Wound Management and Healing

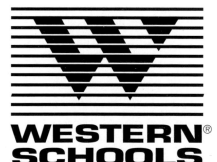

WESTERN® SCHOOLS

By
Janet Stoia Davis, RN, CWOCN
&
Marcia Gay Bales, MSN, MBA, NP-C, CWOCN

ABOUT THE AUTHORS

Janet Stoia Davis, RN, CWOCN, has been a registered nurse since 1976. She graduated from Abbott Northwestern School of Enterostomal Therapy Nursing and became board certified in 1985. Ms. Davis is a partner in Stoia Bales Consultants, a private WOCN firm that contracts its services to managed care, acute care, long-term care, and home health environments; she also performs legal medical review and has been part of various advisory boards related to wound and ostomy care. She is a national lecturer on ostomy, wound, and incontinence issues and has coauthored a video on common perineal skin injuries. Ms. Davis is an active member of the Wound, Ostomy, and Continence Nurses Society (WOCN), and she served several years as chair of their national scholarship committee. Ms. Davis received the ET Nurse of the Year award, Pacific Coast Region of WOCN (PCR/WOCN) 1996, President's Award from PCR/WOCN 2000, and Kaiser Permanente Team Excellence Award, Wound Clinic, 1998.

> **Janet Stoia Davis** has disclosed that she lectures for various wound care companies including Coloplast, 3M, Hollister, ConvaTec and Healthpoint.

Marcia Gay Bales, MSN, MBA, NP-C, CWOCN, has been a registered nurse since 1985. She graduated from the University of California in 1989 with an MBA degree and then attended the University of Southern California School of Enterostomal Therapy Nursing in 1993. Ms. Bales became board certified in 1994 and continues to be board certified in wound, ostomy, and continence care. She attended California State University, received a Master of Science in Nursing – Family Nurse Practitioner in 2002, and currently practices with a family practice physician. She is a partner in Stoia Bales Consultants, a private WOCN firm that contracts its services to managed care, acute care, long-term care, and home health environments. Ms. Bales focuses on the financial aspects of ostomy, wound, and incontinence care. She is an active member of the WOCN and the American Academy of Nurse Practitioners.

> **Marcia Gay Bales** has disclosed that she has no significant financial or other conflicts of interest pertaining to this course book.

ABOUT THE SUBJECT MATTER REVIEWER

Vivian Seide Sternweiler, MS, RN, CWCN, is an experienced clinical nurse specialist, educator, and consultant with specialty certification in wound and skin care management. Her clinical experience as an advanced practice nurse in the metropolitan Boston area has spanned over 15 years. She is currently a clinical nurse specialist for wound and ostomy care at New England Sinai Hospital and Rehabilitation Center in Stoughton, Massachusetts. Ms. Sternweiler has extensive experience in treating an array of wound and skin care conditions, including pressure ulcers, burns, tape tears, and various dermatological conditions. She has presented multiple wound care seminars at a variety of local, regional, and national conferences. In addition, she manages her own consultation practice and participates as a speaker and clinical consultant for such wound care companies as Johnson & Johnson, ConvaTec, and Kinetic Concepts, Inc.

Nurse Planner: Amy Bernard, RN, BSN, MS
Copy Editors: Julie Munden, Jaime Stockslager Buss
Indexer: Sylvia Coates

Western Schools' courses are designed to provide nursing professionals with the educational information they need to enhance their career development. The information provided within these course materials is the result of research and consultation with prominent nursing and medical authorities and is, to the best of our knowledge, current, and accurate. However, the courses and course materials are provided with the understanding that Western Schools is not engaged in offering legal, nursing, medical, or other professional advice.

Western Schools' courses and course materials are not meant to act as a substitute for seeking out professional advice or conducting individual research. When the information provided in the courses and course materials is applied to individual circumstances, all recommendations must be considered in light of the uniqueness pertaining to each situation.

Western Schools' course materials are intended solely for your use and not for the benefit of providing advice or recommendations to third parties. Western Schools devoids itself of any responsibility for adverse consequences resulting from the failure to seek nursing, medical, or other professional advice. Western Schools further devoids itself of any responsibility for updating or revising any programs or publications presented, published, distributed, or sponsored by Western Schools unless otherwise agreed to as part of an individual purchase contract.

Products (including brand names) mentioned or pictured in Western School's courses are not endorsed by Western Schools, the American Nurses Credentialing Center (ANCC) or any state board.

ISBN: 978-1-57801-112-4

IMPORTANT: Read these instructions *BEFORE* proceeding!

Enclosed with your course book, you will find the FasTrax® answer sheet. Use this form to answer all the final exam questions that appear in this course book. If you are completing more than one course, be sure to write your answers on the appropriate answer sheet. Full instructions and complete grading details are printed on the FasTrax instruction sheet, also enclosed with your order. Please review them before starting. *If you are mailing your answer sheet(s) to Western Schools, we recommend you make a copy as a backup.*

ABOUT THIS COURSE

A Pretest is provided with each course to test your current knowledge base regarding the subject matter contained within this course. Your Final Exam is a multiple choice examination. **You will find the exam questions at the end of each chapter.**

Use a black pen to fill in your answer sheet.

A PASSING SCORE

You must score 70% or better in order to pass this course and receive your Certificate of Completion. Should you fail to achieve the required score, we will send you an additional FasTrax answer sheet so that you may make a second attempt to pass the course. Western Schools will allow you three chances to pass the same course...*at no extra charge!* After three failed attempts to pass the same course, your file will be closed.

RECORDING YOUR HOURS

Please monitor the time it takes to complete this course using the handy log sheet on the other side of this page. See below for transferring study hours to the course evaluation.

COURSE EVALUATIONS

In this course book, you will find a short evaluation about the course you are soon to complete. This information is vital to providing Western Schools with feedback on this course. The course evaluation answer section is in the lower right hand corner of the FasTrax answer sheet marked "Evaluation," with answers marked 1–18. Your answers are important to us; please take a few minutes to complete the evaluation.

On the back of the FasTrax instruction sheet, there is additional space to make any comments about the course, the school, and suggested new curriculum. Please mail the FasTrax instruction sheet, with your comments, back to Western Schools in the envelope provided with your course order.

TRANSFERRING STUDY TIME

Upon completion of the course, transfer the total study time from your log sheet to question 18 in the course evaluation. The answers will be in ranges; please choose the proper hour range that best represents your study time. You **MUST** log your study time under question 18 on the course evaluation.

EXTENSIONS

You have two (2) years from the date of enrollment to complete this course. A six (6) month extension may be purchased. If after 30 months from the original enrollment date you do not complete the course, *your file will be closed and no certificate can be issued.*

CHANGE OF ADDRESS?

In the event you have moved during the completion of this course, please call our student services department at 1-800-618-1670, and we will update your file.

A GUARANTEE TO WHICH YOU'LL GIVE HIGH HONORS

If any continuing education course fails to meet your expectations or if you are not satisfied in any manner, for any reason, you may return it for an exchange or a refund (less shipping and handling) within 30 days. Software, video, and audio courses must be returned unopened.

Thank you for enrolling at Western Schools!

WESTERN SCHOOLS
P.O. Box 1930
Brockton, MA 02303
(800) 438-8888
www.westernschools.com

Wound Management and Healing

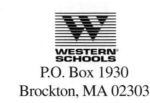

WESTERN® SCHOOLS
P.O. Box 1930
Brockton, MA 02303

Please use this log to total the number of hours you spend reading the text and taking the final examination (use 50-min hours).

Date	Hours Spent
_____	_____
_____	_____
_____	_____
_____	_____
_____	_____
_____	_____
_____	_____
_____	_____
_____	_____
_____	_____
_____	_____
_____	_____
_____	_____

TOTAL ☐

Please log your study hours with submission of your final exam. To log your study time, fill in the appropriate circle under question 18 of the FasTrax® answer sheet under the "Evaluation" section.

Wound Management and Healing

WESTERN SCHOOLS
CONTINUING EDUCATION EVALUATION

Instructions: Mark your answers to the following questions with a black pen on the "Evaluation" section of your FasTrax® answer sheet provided with this course. You should not return this sheet. Please use the scale below to rate the following statements:

A   Agree Strongly   C   Disagree Somewhat
B   Agree Somewhat   D   Disagree Strongly

After completing this course I am able to:

1. Increase knowledge base concerning anatomy and physiology of the skin to include the layers of the skin, the functions of skin, the usual changes that occur with aging, and the relationship of these factors to wound healing.

2. Provide a greater understanding of the basic types of wounds, the usual methods of wound closure, the phases of wound healing, and the relationship wound type and the healing process.

3. Identify systemic and local factors that can impact wound healing and recognize measures that can reduce factors that impede wound repair.

4. State the importance of accurate and timely wound assessment and documentation. Discuss parameters routinely used for wound assessment and documentation and how these factors can be evaluated to assess overall wound repair.

5. Identify the acute surgical wound and factors that affect wound healing, explain care of the incision, recognize abnormalities in the healing process, identify when to follow up with the physician, and present the options for caring for surgical donor sites and basic information on care of surgical flaps and grafts.

6. Discuss factors that place a patient at risk for of skin breakdown and pressure ulcer formation, identify risk assessment tools and how to use them, and present measures to institute to prevent the occurrence of skin breakdown.

7. Identify causes of pressure, anatomical locations for pressure ulcers, aspects of care that need to be included in the treatment plan, and alternative modalities used in pressure ulcer management.

8. Distinguish the most common causes of chronic lower leg ulcers and discuss the treatment and teaching related to each etiology.

9. Discuss the differences between generalized edema and lymphedema, formation of lymphedema, classifications and stages of lymphedema, cornerstone of therapy for lymphedema, and effect of edema on wound management.

10. Identify factors involved in effective wound management, including wound cleansing, infection treatment, debridement, and topical wound care. Discuss principles used to minimize complications and make knowledge-based decisions regarding topical product selection to achieve desired outcomes.

11. Discuss how a wound dressing is removed, applied, and packed in a manner that is least detrimental to the client and discuss the controversy over clean versus sterile technique in changing a wound.

12. Discuss adjunctive therapies that are available for use in the management of wounds and how these therapies can enhance wound resolution.

13. Identify some of the payor sources available for reimbursement of wound care services and steps that can be taken to ensure successful reimbursement.

14. The content of this course was relevant to the objectives.

15. This offering met my professional education needs.

16. The objectives met the overall purpose/goal of the course.

17. The course was generally well written and the subject matter explained thoroughly. (If no, please explain on the back of the FasTrax instruction sheet.)

18. **PLEASE LOG YOUR STUDY HOURS WITH SUBMISSION OF YOUR FINAL EXAM.**
    Please choose the response that best represents the total study hours it took to complete this 30-hour course.

    A. Less than 25 hours   C. 29–32 hours

    B. 25–28 hours   D. Greater than 32 hours

CONTENTS

FIGURES AND TABLES

PRETEST

1. Begin this course by taking the pretest. Circle the answers to the questions on this page, or write the answers on a separate sheet of paper. Do not log answers to the pretest questions on the FasTrax test sheet included with the course.

2. Compare your answers to the PRETEST KEY located in the back of the book. The pretest answer key indicates the course chapter where the content of that question is discussed. Make note of the questions you missed, so that you can focus on those areas as you complete the course.

3. Complete the course by reading each chapter and completing the exam questions at the end of the chapter. Answers to these exam questions should be logged on the FasTrax test sheet included with the course.

1. The pH of normal skin ranges from

    a. 3.5-4.5.

    b. 4.5-5.5.

    c. 5.5-7.0.

    d. 7.0-10.0.

2. The collagen content of adult skin diminishes yearly by

    a. 1%.

    b. 3%.

    c. 4%.

    d. 5%.

3. The phases of wound healing in order are

    a. granulation, epithelialization, and contraction.

    b. proliferative, inflammatory, and differentiation.

    c. inflammatory, proliferative, and differentiation.

    d. inflammatory, granulation, proliferative, and differentiation.

4. The type of wound closure used for a grossly contaminated wound is

    a. primary closure.

    b. secondary closure.

    c. tertiary closure.

    d. flap closure.

5. A systemic factor that affects wound healing is

    a. pressure.

    b. infection.

    c. trauma.

    d. age.

6. A deficiency of carbohydrates leads to

    a. the body using up visceral and muscle proteins for energy.

    b. alteration in taste and anorexia.

    c. increased risk of hemorrhage and hematoma formation.

    d. capillary fragility.

7. Full-thickness skin loss involving damage or necrosis of subcutaneous tissue, which may extend down to, but not through, underlying fascia, is characteristic of a pressure ulcer in

    a. Stage I.
    b. Stage II.
    c. Stage III.
    d. Stage IV.

8. A type of wound that actively generates wound fluid is

    a. black.
    b. red.
    c. yellow.
    d. white.

9. A method of documenting a two-dimensional wound size is

    a. foam dressings.
    b. wound tracings.
    c. wound molds.
    d. fluid instillation.

10. Yellow or brown tissue in a wound bed indicates

    a. nonviable tissue.
    b. infection.
    c. viable tissue.
    d. healing tissue.

11. The subscales of the Braden scale include

    a. mobility, incontinence, physical condition, activity, and mental state.
    b. mobility, friction, shear, activity, and mental state.
    c. sensory perception, incontinence, activity, and mental state.
    d. sensory perception, skin moisture, activity, mobility, nutritional intake, and friction and shear.

12. Patients who have been seated and cannot reposition themselves should be returned to their beds after

    a. 30 minutes.
    b. 1 hour.
    c. 1 hour, 30 minutes.
    d. 2 hours.

13. The type of pressure relief that an egg crate mattress offers is

    a. static air.
    b. high-density foam support.
    c. comfort only.
    d. low-air-loss therapy.

14. A noninvasive adjunctive therapy that uses electrical waveforms to promote wound healing is known as

    a. electrical stimulation.
    b. ultrasound.
    c. hyperbaric oxygen.
    d. cultured epithelium.

15. An adequate choice for compression therapy in a patient with venous disease would be

    a. antiembolism stockings.
    b. ace wraps.
    c. therapeutic support stockings.
    d. gauze roll.

16. The most common reason a plantar ulcer in a patient with diabetes does not heal is

    a. poor circulation.
    b. intermittent loss of glucose control.
    c. lack of pressure relief.
    d. infection.

17. A classic characteristic of arterial ulcers is

    a. high amount of exudate.

    b. nonpainful, often necrotic.

    c. location on the plantar surface of the foot.

    d. a deep, pale, or necrotic wound bed.

18. The edema associated with venous stasis ulcers usually is a result of

    a. high-protein fluid in the interstitial spaces.

    b. water and body fluids in the interstitial spaces.

    c. salt retention.

    d. improper performance of ankle and foot exercises.

19. A superficial partial-thickness wound could be treated with

    a. a wet-to-dry dressing.

    b. a hydrocolloid.

    c. a transparent film.

    d. an enzyme.

20. Antibiotic therapy should be used in the treatment of chronic wounds that have

    a. thick, yellow-tan drainage.

    b. increased odor.

    c. a positive wound culture.

    d. nonhealing qualities.

21. The psi that is safe and effective in wound irrigation is

    a. 4–15 psi.

    b. 8 psi only.

    c. 2–10 psi.

    d. 25 psi only.

22. Which of the following statements is correct?

    a. Pressure ulcer dressings should be sterile.

    b. Dressing removal should be quick to avoid pain.

    c. Care should be taken to eliminate trauma to surrounding skin.

    d. If any portion of a dressing adheres to the wound bed, it should be removed slowly to traumatize only the top layer of the wound bed.

23. A patient with a large diabetic foot ulcer who is receiving antibiotics for osteomyelitis would be appropriate for treatment with

    a. growth factors only.

    b. growth factors or vacuum-assisted closure.

    c. vacuum-assisted closure, growth factors, or bioengineered skin.

    d. electrical stimulation or bioengineered skin only.

24. The way health care is delivered in the home health and skilled nursing areas has been impacted most by

    a. Medicare.

    b. Medicaid/MediCal.

    c. health maintenance organizations.

    d. Balanced Budget Act.

INTRODUCTION

The evaluation and treatment of wounds is a critical component of a patient's care and recovery. An understanding of the current concepts in wound management provides the clinician with the needed information for optimal outcomes. With all of the products that are available, wound management can seem like a complicated task. When the constraints on reimbursement are added and available resources are evaluated, wound management becomes a continuing challenge for health care clinicians. Knowing the brand names of products or how they are applied is not enough for success at wound healing. A fundamental knowledge of the different types of wounds, their etiologies, factors of exacerbation or improvement, wound healing physiology, and accepted standards of treatment lends greater success to the clinician who practices with these principles. In addition, wound management is a multidisciplinary team approach. Collaboration with colleagues can help dictate appropriate and individualized care for each patient.

Although a multidisciplinary approach is needed for optimizing outcomes, nursing personnel are commonly the primary providers of direct patient care and, therefore, play an important role in wound management. Clinicians need to be informed of methods to promote healing and assist the client's family and caregivers with available resources to do the same. We still believe that this concept is true and that the nursing profession is responsible for the day-to-day care and management of a patient's wound care needs. This statement from Levine (1973) still lends support for that thought: "Every healing process, regardless of its nature, occurs over a period of time. The success of the ultimate healing depends in large measure on what happens to the individual during that time. The nurse is the person on the health team who shares the most time with the patient, and thus no worker can influence the success of the healing process more than the nurse. Nursing processes of every kind are dedicated to the promotion of healing."

This course book consists of 13 chapters. Chapter 1 describes normal anatomy and physiology of the skin. Chapter 2 discusses the physiology of wound healing. Chapter 3 relates many of the factors that exert an effect on wound healing. Chapter 4 gives details on accurate assessment and documentation of wounds so that the treatment plan can be evaluated for outcomes. Chapter 5 begins a discussion on the different types of wounds and details acute surgical wounds. The chapter also discusses the management of flaps, grafts, and donor sites. Chapter 6 describes risk assessment and prevention of pressure ulcers. Chapter 7 discusses pressure ulcers in more detail. Chapter 8 looks at lower extremity ulcers, including venous, arterial, and neuropathic ulcers. Chapter 9 offers information on the effects of edema on wound management and provides some suggestions on how to manage edema. Chapter 10 evaluates patient management issues, such as infection control, debridement, and moist wound healing. In addition, it outlines various types of wound dressings, including their actions, indications, advantages, and disadvantages. Chapter 11 describes the basic dressing change procedure and discusses aspects of the procedure that are fundamental in wound care. Chapter 12 discusses adjunctive wound care therapies that show promise in improving wound healing outcomes. Chapter 13 provides information pertinent to reimbursement issues with regard to wound management.

This course book is designed for clinicians from various health care disciplines, such as nurses, physical therapists, occupational therapists, dietitians, physician assistants, nurse practitioners, and physicians who are new to the management of wounds. We wrote this course to give the clinician an insight into the fundamental aspects of wound healing and treatment so that an optimal outcome can be achieved. This course book was not developed with the intent of providing the clinician with every current wound product and use, every wound treatment modality available, or the most advanced wound care research; rather, it was designed to provide a fundamental knowledge of what needs to be considered with wound management. We hope that at the end of the course, the clinician will have obtained this information and will have a greater appreciation of what resources are needed for effective wound healing. We also hope that the clinician will recognize that the management of wounds requires a multifaceted approach in which several factors are evaluated before implementation of a treatment plan. Wound management in today's health care arena has advanced to a more aggressive level, and additional readings and courses are necessary for clinicians to be knowledgeable in these advanced treatment modalities.

Janet Stoia Davis
Marcia Gay Bales

CHAPTER 1

ANATOMY AND PHYSIOLOGY OF THE SKIN

CHAPTER OBJECTIVE

Upon completion of the chapter, the reader will have an increased knowledge base concerning anatomy and physiology of the skin to include the layers of the skin, the functions of skin, the usual changes that occur with aging, and the relationship of these factors to wound healing.

LEARNING OBJECTIVES

After completion of the chapter, the reader will be able to

1. identify the layers of the epidermis and their functions.

2. state the components and the cells of the dermis and their functions.

3. list three changes that occur in the skin with age.

4. state how the health of the skin affects the wound healing process.

INTRODUCTION

Weighing between 6 and 8 pounds, the skin, (also known as the cutis or integument), is the largest organ of the human body. It covers an area of more than 20 square feet in an average-sized adult and is composed of two layers, the epidermis and the dermis. The skin allows the body to interface with the rest of the world and is an extremely important psychological factor in a person's well-being. Cosmetic appearance of the skin plays a major fac-

tor in modern society, which places importance on beauty. Skin that is damaged from scarring, wounds, or other imperfections can affect a person's emotional well-being (Maklebust & Sieggreen, 2001).

The appearance and texture of skin depends on regional differences in blood flow, glandular distribution, and amount of hair. The appearance and thickness of skin also varies with anatomical location. Skin can range in thickness from 1/50 of an inch over the eyelids to 1/3 of an inch over the palms of the hands and the soles of the feet. The pH of skin ranges from 4.5-5.5 and serves as the protective acid mantle to maintain the normal skin flora. The skin is an extremely sensitive indicator of overall health, both physical and emotional, and can tell a lot about the individual and the ability for wound healing. Clinicians who are involved in the promotion of healthy skin maintenance and assistance with wound healing benefit from basic knowledge of the anatomy and physiology of the skin and of general skin functions (Maklebust & Sieggreen, 2001).

STRUCTURE OF THE SKIN

The skin consists of two main structures (see Figure 1-1). The outer layer, the epidermis, is composed of epithelial cells; whereas the inner layer, the dermis, is composed of connective tissue. The epidermis and dermis are separated by the basement membrane. The epidermis is made up of stratified squamous epithelium with keratinization and its layers vary in cell shape, size, and structure. The dermis, which has a dense connective tissue

FIGURE 1-1
Layers of the Skin

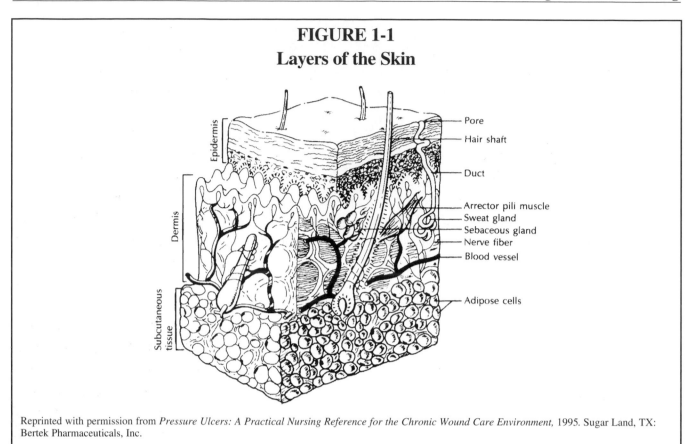

Reprinted with permission from *Pressure Ulcers: A Practical Nursing Reference for the Chronic Wound Care Environment,* 1995. Sugar Land, TX: Bertek Pharmaceuticals, Inc.

composition, is supported underneath by a loose connective tissue called the hypodermis, or subcutis, that allows for movement of the skin (Bryant, 2000; Maklebust & Sieggreen, 2001; Milne, Corbett, & Dubuc, 2003).

Epidermis

The epidermis is avascular and consists of five layers. These layers, starting with the outermost layer, are the stratum corneum, stratum lucidum, stratum granulosum, stratum spinosum, and stratum germinativum. The epidermis is constantly being renewed, with a cellular turnover rate every 26–42 days. Complete epidermal renewal ranges from 45–75 days.

Stratum Corneum. The stratum corneum, also referred to as the horny layer, is the tough, outer layer of the epidermis that consists of dead keratinized cells. These cells allow the skin to withstand the daily rigors of mechanical and chemical trauma, such as hand washing, bathing, scratching, and exercising. The keratin

in these cells is a tough, insoluble protein that resists changes in temperature or pH as well as the chemical digestion of trypsin and pepsin. Keratin is the same protein found in the hair and nails.

Stratum Lucidum. This layer is transparent in nature, is usually one to five cells thick, and is seen where the epidermis is thicker. It is present where more stresses are noted, such as the palms of the hands and the soles of the feet, yet absent in thinner-skinned areas such as the eyelids. This layer tends to be transparent and is often difficult to distinguish histologically. The stratum lucidum is considered a transitional layer that contains active lysosomal enzymes that degrade the nucleus and additional organelles of cells prior to moving into the stratum corneum.

Stratum Granulosum. This layer is also one to five cells thick. It has protein-type granules in its keratinocytes that can be intensely stained with acidic and basic dyes. These cells are diamond shaped and have a protein in their granules that helps to organize the keratin filaments in the intracellular space. The stratum granulosum is a metabolically active layer that contains both active keratinocytes and Langerhans' cells. Langerhans' cells originate in the bone marrow but migrate to all areas of the body, including the skin. These cells play a major role in immune reaction and affect the inflammatory phase of allergic contact dermatitis. These specialized cells participate in immunologic responses functioning in the antigen recognition and processing areas. These cells also act as macrophages ingesting potential antigenic compounds to prevent the allergic component. Langerhans' cells are susceptible to ultraviolet light and are easily damaged by this radiation. This relationship may be an important aspect of the pathogenesis of sunlight-induced skin malignancy.

Stratum Spinosum. This layer of the epidermis is referred to as the prickly layer because of the appearance of the cytoplasmic structures within the cells. The prominent features of the stratum spinosum are cells called desmosomes that form a type of cell-cell junction. The stratum spinosum may be considered part of the underlying basal cell layer, yet it cannot regenerate. The stratum spinosum contains a large number of Langerhans' cells as well.

Stratum Germinativum. This innermost layer of the epidermis is also referred to as the basal layer, or stratum basale. It is composed of one layer of mitotically active cells called basal cells, or basal keratinocytes. This single layer of cells is the only layer of epidermis that can regenerate. The other cells that do not regenerate are repaired by scar formation. The basal cells' migration to the skin's surface can take 2–3 weeks. As they move upward, they start the process of differentiation. Several structures, called rete ridges, protrude downward from the basal layer into the dermis. These ridges help

anchor the epidermis to the dermis. Another important cell in the basal layer is the melanocyte, which gives the skin its pigmentation. The number of melanocytes in normal skin is the same regardless of skin color. There is approximately 1 melanocyte for every 36 basal cells. The main differences between light-colored skin and dark-colored skin are the size and the distribution of the melanosomes and the activity of the melanocytes. Melanosomes are the structures that contain the melanin pigment. The yellow pigment that is seen in some individuals is due to carotene or carotenoids. Melanocytes that have not been injured produce melanin at a steady rate to provide continual protection of cellular DNA from ultraviolet radiation. Ultraviolet radiation increases skin pigmentation by two mechanisms: 1) photooxidation of existing melanin and 2) delay of new melanin production due to the process of tanning. The melanocytes eventually migrate into keratinocytes in the basal layer and are degraded by intracellular lysosomal enzymes as the process of keratinocyte migration continues toward the stratum corneum (Bryant, 2000; Maklebust & Sieggreen, 2001).

Basement Membrane Zone

The basement membrane zone separates the epidermis from the dermis and is commonly referred to as the dermoepidermal junction. This junction helps to provide structural support and allows exchange of fluids and cells between the dermis and the epidermis. The rete ridges from the epidermis interface with the upward projections of the papillary dermis, locking together to help prevent the epidermis from sliding back and forth. As the aging process progresses, the dermoepidermal junction flattens, causing the area of contact between the dermis and the epidermis to diminish by one-third. This dermoepidermal separation places the geriatric population at greater risk for skin tears and other skin injuries. The basement membrane zone is the layer of skin that is affected in blister formation. When wound healing is taking place, the basement membrane zone is disrupted and requires reforming (Bryant, 2000; Maklebust & Sieggreen, 2001).

Dermis

The dermis, which lies directly below the epidermis, supplies nutrition and support for the epidermis. Also called the corium, the dermis is the thickest tissue layer of the skin. The thickness ranges from 2–4 mm depending on the area of the body. For example, the dermis on an individual's back is thicker than the dermis that covers the scalp, abdomen, forehead, thigh, palm, and wrist.

The dermis is a strong, extracellular matrix composed of collagen and elastic fibers that provides the skin with mechanical strength. It has two layers of connective tissue that contain blood vessels, nerves, and integumentary appendages, such as hair, nails, and the sweat glands. The most important cell of the dermis is the fibroblast, which has many functions. Fibroblasts produce collagen, elastin, and ground substance. Collagen is a protein that gives skin its mechanical strength. Elastic fibers (elastin) are synthesized to give the skin stretch and flexibility. The ground substance helps to cushion and lubricate.

The two layers of the dermis are the papillary dermis and the reticular dermis. The papillary dermis is the outermost layer and is formed of collagen and reticular fibers that are important to healing. This layer of the dermis also has a supply of capillaries that provide nourishment to the epidermis and appendages. The reticular dermis is the inner layer. It is made up of thicker networks of collagen bundles that help to anchor the skin to the subcutaneous tissue. These thicker fibers assist with increased elasticity (Maklebust & Sieggreen, 2001).

Subcutaneous Tissue and Fascia

The subcutaneous tissue, sometimes referred to as the hypodermis, lies just below the dermis. It is composed of adipose tissue that houses major blood vessels, nerves, and lymphatics. It functions as a heat insulator, nutrition supplier, and mechanical shock absorber. This cushioning effect also assists in the mobility of the skin over underlying structures. The subcutaneous tissue attaches the dermis to underlying structures.

Below the subcutaneous layer is the superficial fascia. The superficial fascia is a type of dense, firm membranous connective tissue that covers muscles, blood vessels, and nerves. Fascial layers vary in function, thickness, and strength depending upon where the fascia is located. The deep fascia is less elastic and forms a sheath or envelope-like covering for the muscles, nerves, and blood vessels (Bryant, 2000; Maklebust & Sieggreen, 2001).

FUNCTIONS OF THE SKIN

The skin has several important functions that it carries out on a daily basis. These functions include protection, thermoregulation, sensation, metabolism, and communication.

Protection

The skin acts as a protective mechanism against many types of insults, including chemical, mechanical, bacterial, and viral. It protects the body from ultraviolet radiation as well as from excessive fluid and electrolyte losses. The skin helps the body maintain a homeostatic environment. Protection from mechanical insults comes mainly from the fibroelastic tissue of the dermis, which consists of collagen and elastin. Collagen, which is the most abundant protein in mammals, comprises 25% of total weight and provides the tensile strength that allows the skin to resist tearing forces. Elastin is found within collagen but in smaller amounts. Larger concentrations of elastin are found in the blood vessels (Bryant, 2000). The stratum corneum, along with secretions from the sebaceous glands and the skin's immune system, provides excellent protection from a variety of insults. Keratin, the insoluble protein in the stratum corneum, is a main component of this defense. The constant shedding of cells from the stratum corneum also prevents damage from microorganisms. The sebum that is secreted onto the skin from the hair follicles provides an acidic coating with a mean pH of 5.5, which serves as an effective barrier and retards the growth of microorganisms. Finally, normal skin flora provides resistance to pathogenic microorganisms by bacterial interference. Protection from ultraviolet light is achieved by melanin that forms skin pigmentation. Individuals who have an increased amount, distribution, or synthesis of melanin tend to have greater protection from ultraviolet radiation (Bryant, 2000).

Thermoregulation

The skin provides a barrier between the outside and inside environments that helps to maintain body temperature via thermoregulation. Thermoregulation of the body occurs by means of circulation and sweating. Blood vessels either dilate to dissipate heat or constrict to contain heat and supply it to other organs. When blood vessels dilate, blood flow is increased and heat is released by means of conduction, radiation, convection, and evaporation. Vasoconstriction, on the other hand, keeps heat in to be sent to other organs for use. For humans, the act of shivering is another important method of maintaining warmth. Sweating occurs when the eccrine glands increase activity. These glands are found abundantly on the palms of the hands and soles of the feet and are mainly under the control of the nervous system. They respond to changes in temperature or emotion (Bryant, 2000).

Sensation

The function of sensation comes from nerve receptors in the skin. These receptors are sensitive to pain, touch, temperature, and pressure. When nerve receptors are stimulated, they transmit impulses to the cerebral cortex for interpretation. The resultant combinations of these sensations are interpreted as a form of burning, tickling, or itching. The skin's sensation abilities are part of the body's integrative response to adapt to and protect itself from the surrounding environment. Sensation works with the function of regulation. The signals received from the skin, sensation, signals the body to regulate. The regulation occurs by various means: sweat, shivering, weight shifts of the body, scratching, or laughter. The importance of touch has been demonstrated in interaction with infants and children. Deprivation of the touch sensation has been linked to psychomotor retardation and an increased risk of mortality (Bryant, 2000; Milne, Corbett, & Dubuc, 2003).

Metabolism

The skin also assists with some forms of metabolism. For example, vitamin D is synthesized in the presence of sunlight. Ultraviolet radiation converts a sterol, 7-dehydrocholesterol to cholecalciferol, vitamin D. Vitamin D helps in the metabolism of calcium and phosphate and is important in the mineralization of bone.

Communication

Human skin also functions as a means of communication and identification. The skin acts as the organ of nonverbal communication. Looking at a person's face identifies that person and allows a method of judging internal and external beauty. Injury to the skin can alter functional and physiological sensation as well as change a person's body image. Scarring can lead to changes in everyday life, from clothing changes to avoidance of public exposure. These changes many times lead to decreased self-esteem. Communication involving facial skin and underlying muscles also occurs via expressions, such as smiling, frowning, and laughing. Finally, the skin plays another important role in human communication, specifically, providing such feelings as comfort, love, and friendship via touch (Bryant, 2000; Maklebust & Sieggreen, 2001; Milne, Corbett, & Dubuc, 2003).

SKIN CHANGES ASSOCIATED WITH AGING

As aging occurs, many skin changes take place that can affect tissue injury and repair:

• reduced dermal proteins lead to increased fluid loss,

• increased epidermal rate of turnover leads to a decrease in skin moisture content,

• decreased number of sweat glands and sebum causes a decrease in the bacteriostatic ability of the skin,

• degeneration of elastin leads to wrinkles,

• thinning of the dermoepidermal junction causes skin to become less pliable and more prone to skin tears and other injuries from trauma,

• general thinning of the epidermis leads to an increased risk of skin tears with minimal trauma,

• changes in capillary loop structure leads to bruising,

• a reduction in the number of Langerhans' cells and mast cells leads to a decreased inflammatory response and impaired wound healing, and

• changes in the sebum chemical composition tends to decrease the bacteriostatic properties of the skin

(Milne, Corbett, & Dubuc, 2003).

In addition to these changes, the number of sweat glands diminishes with age and atrophy and thinning of both the fatty and epithelial layers of the skin occurs. The amount of subcutaneous fat on the lower legs and forearms in older individuals is diminished, further exposing the bony prominences and leading to risk of injury. Skin changes are due to a progressive destruction of the architecture of the dermal connective tissue. Because dermal fibroblasts are one of the few cells of the body that possess a finite number of replications, usually 50 to 100 in a lifetime, they cease to replicate in the older individual. Furthermore, collagen and elastin undergo degenerative changes that make their fibers shrink. The collagen content of skin has been shown to diminish by approximately 1% per year throughout adult life. The combination of these changes leads to thin, dry, and inelastic skin. The dermoepidermal junction weakens as well, increasing the tendency of the epidermis to slide over the dermis with minor friction or shearing forces causing skin tears and other abrasions (Maklebust & Sieggreen, 2001).

It is not uncommon for older individuals to complain of dry, itchy skin as well as being cold. This may be attributed to the loss of subcutaneous tissue. A change in the number of melanocytes results in skin pallor and whitening of Caucasian skin and graying of the hair. The loss of hair in general and the presence of wrinkles also accompany aging as permanent infoldings of the epithelium and subepithelium take place. The aging individual also tends to lose body hair and develop wrinkles. Repeated stress on the skin with facial changes tends to be a large factor in the formation of facial wrinkles. However, the most important factor that affects the formation of wrinkles and additional age-related skin changes is exposure to the sun.

These age-related changes make apparent the need for additional care for prevention and treatment of wound occurrence with aging skin. The fragile skin of an older adult requires a more gentle approach to care. Gentle cleansing with warm water only is usually sufficient for daily skin hygiene. Friction with cleansing should be minimized with soft cloths and patting the skin dry versus rubbing or scrubbing the area. Gentle cleansers should also be used instead of more caustic substances. Moisturizing the skin is always an important component of overall skin health (Maklebust & Sieggreen, 2001).

SUMMARY

As the largest of the organ systems, the integumentary system serves many body functions, including protection, thermoregulation, sensation, metabolism, and communication. The status of the skin can tell a lot about the overall health of an individual. It is composed of two layers, the epidermis and the dermis. The epidermis is made up of specialized epithelial cells; the dermis is composed of connective tissue. Each of these layers has its own specialized cells that help with skin functions. Keratinocytes in the epidermis help protect against chemical and mechanical trauma, and fibroblasts in the dermis make elastin and collagen, which give the skin its strength and elasticity. With aging, the components of skin change, making it more vulnerable to outside forces and leading to increased injury and delayed healing. Understanding the composition of the skin layers, the specialized cells within these layers, and the cells' functions assists the clinician with monitoring the wound healing process. Knowing skin changes that occur with aging can help the clinician offer appropriate prevention measures and treatment modalities that will reduce the potential for skin injury as well as promote healing for those individuals who have been injured.

EXAM QUESTIONS

CHAPTER 1
Questions 1-7

1. The skin layer that contains connective tissue is the
   a. epidermis.
   b. dermis.
   c. subcutaneous tissue.
   d. basement membrane zone.

2. The layer of the epidermis that is referred to as the "basal layer" is the
   a. stratum lucidum.
   b. stratum granulosum.
   c. stratum spinosum.
   d. stratum germinativum.

3. The layer of the epidermis that allows skin to withstand mechanical and chemical trauma is the
   a. stratum corneum.
   b. stratum lucidum.
   c. stratum germinativum.
   d. stratum spinosum.

4. The change that takes place in the basement membrane zone with aging is
   a. widening of the dermoepidermal junction.
   b. flattening of the subcutaneous layer.
   c. increasing secretions of the sweat glands.
   d. flattening of the dermoepidermal junction.

5. The most important cell of the dermis is the
   a. macrophage.
   b. fibroblast.
   c. leukocyte.
   d. red blood cell.

6. Collagen affects wound healing by providing
   a. stretch and flexibility.
   b. mechanical strength.
   c. utilization of nutrients.
   d. binding at the basement membrane.

7. A normal skin change that occurs with aging is
   a. increased collagen production.
   b. decreased need for skin moisturizers.
   c. general thinning of the epidermis.
   d. decreased need for sun protection.

CHAPTER 2

THE PHYSIOLOGY OF WOUND HEALING

CHAPTER OBJECTIVES

Upon completion of the chapter, the reader will have a greater understanding of the basic types of wounds, usual methods of wound closure, the phases of wound healing, and the relationships between wound types and the healing process.

LEARNING OBJECTIVES

After completion of the chapter, the reader will be able to

1. describe two types of wounds.
2. state the three classifications of wound closure.
3. state the three phases of wound healing.
4. discuss the physiology of the wound phases.

INTRODUCTION

There are different ways that an individual can receive a wound or become wounded — by surgical means, pressure-related causes, vascular means, and trauma to name a few. The wound may be closed immediately, as with a surgical intervention, or the wound may be allowed to close on its own. The healing process for each of these etiologies tends to follow a particular healing trajectory. Understanding the phases of this healing trajectory and the factors that affect healing allows the clinician to judge whether a wound is progressing as it should and what measures, if any, need to be instituted to improve the healing outcome.

TYPES OF WOUNDS

There are several types of wounds and factors that contribute to the development of a wound. General categories of wound types include acute, chronic, surgical, nonsurgical, pressure, vascular, traumatic, partial or full thickness, laceration, diabetic or neuropathic, and burn related. Factors that routinely affect these types of wounds include pressure, friction, shearing, moisture, cold, trauma, radiation, heat, malignancy, ischemia, vasculitic injury, factitious injury, and chemical contact. These types of wounds and common factors are explored in more detail throughout the remaining chapters (Milne, Corbett, & Dubuc, 2003).

WOUND CLOSURE

When an individual develops a wound, how will it heal or close? Wound closure classifications are based on the amount of tissue loss that is present. The amount of tissue loss determines the projected time of healing, the amount of granulation or scar formation to be noted, and the length of time necessary for contraction to close the wound. Three basic classifications of wound closure are used in wound healing studies: primary, secondary, and tertiary wound closure or healing.

Primary Closure

Primary, or first intention, wound closure or healing is possible when wound edges are immediately approximated after the injury. Primary wound closure allows for epithelialization within 72 hours. The wound usually has minimal or little tissue loss upon closure. An example of primary wound closure is immediate closure of a surgical wound (see Figures 2-1 through 2-3). Primary closure minimizes the volume of connective tissue deposition that is required for wound repair and closure and restores the epithelium, which functions as a barrier for infection. Wound healing proceeds under the normal healing trajectory, which usually means that these wounds heal quickly with minimal scar formation, unless infection or other factors disrupt the process. Some wounds cannot be managed by primary closure due to edema or infection. These wounds are either left open to be healed by secondary intention or are left open to treat the immediate problems and then later closed. The latter is called delayed primary closure (Bryant, 2000).

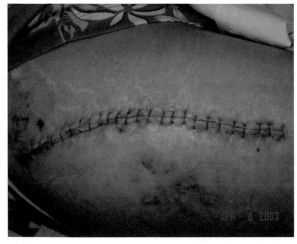

FIGURE 2-1
Primary Closure
Right Hip Incision

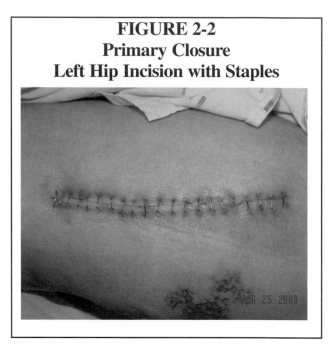

FIGURE 2-2
Primary Closure
Left Hip Incision with Staples

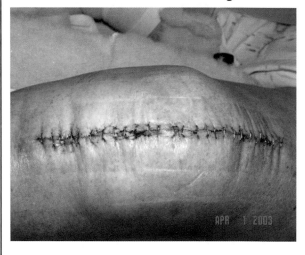

FIGURE 2-3
Primary Closure
Knee Incision with Staples

Secondary Closure

Secondary intention wound closure healing takes place when wound edges are left open and unopposed. Secondary closure allows for treatment of necrotic and grossly contaminated wounds, wounds with edema, and wounds that have additional factors that prevent closure. Wounds closed by secondary intention heal more slowly due to a larger defect that must be filled (see Figure 2-4). Granulation tissue forms in the wound base and fills in the defect. The wound usually continues to close with granulation tissue filling the wound and contraction of the wound margins occuring. When bacterial counts are low, these wounds may also be closed surgically, either by approximation of the wound edges or through the use of skin grafting. Because these wounds are left open and the epithelial barrier is not present, these wounds are more susceptible to microorganisms and to infection. Such wounds as pressure ulcers, vascular ulcers, diabetic or neuropathic ulcers, and wounds secondary to abscess formation are allowed to heal by secondary intention. Due to the time it takes for these wounds to heal, they tend to be classified as chronic wounds, and they require excellent follow-through by wound care clinicians to optimize healing outcomes (Bryant, 2000).

FIGURE 2-4
Abdominal Wound Status/Post
Tummy Tuck

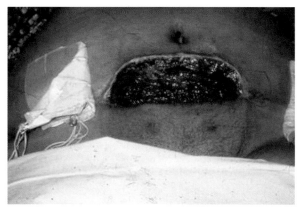

Tertiary Closure

Tertiary, or third intention, wound closure healing is seen with delayed primary closure. Delayed primary closure is utilized when a wound with a low-grade bacterial contamination, edema, or some other immediate factor is left open for observation and treatment. When the infection, necrosis, or edema is resolved the wound edges can be approximated. Abdominal surgical wounds tend to close in this fashion. The wound usually continues on a nor-

mal healing trajectory similar to that of primary closure (Bryant, 2000).

ACUTE VERSUS
CHRONIC WOUNDS

It is difficult to define acute and chronic wounds. Wounds are usually described as acute or chronic based upon the time it takes for them to fully heal. An acute wound, as its name implies, begins to heal rather abruptly. Trauma and surgery tend to be the main etiologies for acute wounds. Chronic wounds, on the other hand, heal at a much slower rate and tend to be the pressure or vascular ulcer type. Regardless of the wound type or severity, there are two main mechanisms for healing or repair: 1) regeneration of damaged or lost tissue with the same type of tissue or 2) connective tissue repair, in which the damaged or lost tissue is replaced with scar formation. Connective tissue repair is a less satisfactory method of repair because normal function and appearance may not be maintained. The mechanism for repair and healing depends on the tissue layers involved and their capacity for regeneration. The healing process for partial-thickness and full-thickness wounds describes these repair processes (Bryant, 2000).

WOUND HEALING
CONCEPTS

- A wound disrupts the normal anatomic structure and function of a tissue.

- Acute wound repair proceeds through an orderly and timely process, with the end result being sustained restoration of anatomic and functional integrity.

- Chronic wound repair fails to proceed through an orderly and timely process that produces functional and anatomic integrity, or the repair proceeds through the healing process but the functional and anatomic outcome is not sustained.

- Wound healing is considered a dynamic process with an end outcome of restoration of anatomic continuity and function.

- Orderly wound healing is a sequence of inflammation, angiogenesis, tissue matrix regeneration, contraction, epithelialization, and remodeling.

- Timely wound healing depends upon the etiology of the wound and varies with the unique characteristics of the wound and the individual's internal and external environments.

- A wound is considered ideally healed when it returns to a normal anatomic structure, function, and appearance.

- A wound is considered acceptably healed when it sustains functional and anatomic continuity.

- A wound is considered minimally healed when it reaches anatomic continuity without a sustained functional result and is subject to recurrence in the future.

(Maklebust & Sieggreen, 2001)

THE WOUND HEALING PROCESS

When the body is wounded, it responds with a cascade of events that lead to a reparative process. The cascade of wound healing events depends upon whether a wound is partial or full thickness. Partial-thickness wound healing occurs in wounds that involve epidermal loss and possibly partial loss of the dermis. The repair process for this type of wound is regeneration, with the key mediator being the epithelial cell. Repair consists of epithelial proliferation and lateral migration or resurfacing as well as reestablishment of normal skin layers and function. When the dermis is involved, connective tissue repair takes place along with epithelialization.

Full-thickness wounds involve total loss of the epidermal and dermal layers with injury into at least the subcutaneous tissue. The wound may even extend deeper into the underlying muscle, bone, or other supporting structures. Repair for this type of wound consists of scar formation that includes connective tissue repair. The three phases of wound repair for a full-thickness wound are the inflammatory, proliferative, and maturation phases. Full-thickness wound healing is a complicated process, and the phases of healing often overlap. Full-thickness wounds can be complicated by necrosis, infection, sinus tracts, or undermining (Bryant, 2000).

Inflammatory Phase

The inflammatory, or defensive, phase begins when the initial wounding insult activates the tissue repair cascade and starts local vasoconstriction, which lasts approximately 5–10 minutes. A chemical reaction drives multiple cells into the wounded area to defend and revitalize the injured tissue. Platelets initially respond, depositing granules for clotting and stimulation of growth factors. The granules assist with fibrin deposition and clot formation to seal the wound.

Vasodilation leads to vascular permeability, allowing leakage of neutrophils into the wounded space. The inflammation that occurs is caused by enzymes, fluid, and proteins, that become trapped in the extracellular space. Leukocytes, or white blood cells, migrate to the area and begin digesting organic debris. The white blood cells recede in 24 hours as monocytes migrate to the wound. The monocytes turn into macrophages, which are key to the healing process. These cells assist with wound debridement, fibroplasia management, and degradation of collagen. They also release an angiogenic factor that stimulates new blood vessel growth and a growth factor that is responsible for fibroblast and collagen synthesis. Local erythema, edema, and tenderness of the surrounding tissues clinically characterize the inflammatory phase. The main functions of the inflammatory phase are to start the wound healing cascade, remove debris from the area, and prepare the wound for regeneration of new tissue (Bryant, 2000; Maklebust & Sieggreen, 2001; Milne, Corbet, & Dubuc, 2003).

Proliferative Phase

The proliferative, or fibroblastic, phase of wound healing begins approximately 3–4 days after the initial wounding and lasts for about 15–16 days. During this phase, the main reparative functions include deposition of connective tissue and collagen cross-linking. The most notable events of the proliferative phase are granulation, epithelialization, and contraction of the wound. Fibroblasts are the most important cells during this phase; they have the task of multiplying and synthesizing collagen, which fills in the wound and provides strength. While collagen is being produced, new capillaries form by budding from nearby vessels. These then grow into the wound, grow into loops and nourish the new tissue. These new capillary loops give a red granular appearance to the wound bed, hence the name, granulation tissue. This granulation tissue provides a good defense against surface contamination.

Epithelialization, the next event in the proliferative phase, transpires as the epithelial cells from the wound margins migrate across the wound surface to seal the wound. Wounds that fall under the primary healing category show fibrin deposition in a few hours and epithelialization in 1–2 days. Secondary healing wounds have rapid epithelial migration initially, however, migration slows and weeks may pass before the process is complete. When a scab or hard eschar is present over the wound, the epithelial cells must go under the scab, delaying wound closure. New epithelial tissue at this stage remains extremely fragile.

The final event of the proliferative phase is contraction of the wound, which begins about 5 days after the initial wounding. The myofibroblast is the cell responsible for contraction. Myofibroblasts are special cells that exhibit contractility and collagen synthesis. The contraction of scar tissue occurs as

the wound decreases in size by movement of the surrounding tissue toward the center of the initial wound (Bryant, 2000; Maklebust & Sieggreen, 2001; Milne, Corbett, & Dubuc, 2003).

Differentiation Phase

The differentiation, or maturation, phase is the remodeling phase of wound healing. It is the longest phase. This is the time during which the collagen in the wound undergoes repeated degradation and resynthesis. It begins around day 21 and differs in length, depending on what type of wound is present. For primary healing wounds, maximum total collagen is usually completed by day 42. Equilibrium between collagen synthesis and collagen breakdown is reached at this time. The scar that is formed continues to gain tensile strength for 2 years. During days 1–14, the new tissues develop approximately 30%–50% of the original fiber strength and continue to progress until final tensile strength (80%) is reached. The skin over a wound never returns to its prewound tensile strength and, therefore, wounds are at risk for future injury (Maklebust & Sieggreen, 2001).

SUMMARY

The etiology of a wound may be related to surgery, pressure, trauma, or some other means, yet the process of wound repair will usually go through some type of healing progression. Wounds that are classified as acute usually progress to closure along an orderly healing trajectory. Wounds that do not follow an orderly and timely healing trajectory are classified as chronic.

Wound closure is classified as either primary, secondary, or tertiary closure, depending on the type of wound and any necrosis, infection, or other factors that need to be treated. Partial-thickness wounds heal by epithelial migration; whereas full-thickness wounds heal by granulation tissue filling in the defect and re-epithelialization. When full thickness wounds undergo wound repair, three healing phases come into play — the inflammatory, proliferative, and differentiation phases. The inflammatory phase activates the tissue repair cascade, removes necrotic debris, and prepares the wound for tissue regeneration. The proliferative phase is marked by the deposition of connective tissue and collagen cross-linking. The formation of granulation tissue, epithelial migration, and wound contraction are the main events of the proliferative phase. The differentiation, or maturation, phase of wound healing takes place as collagen undergoes remodeling to increase its strength. The significance of the wound healing phases is that they set a timeline along which wound healing proceeds. If the timeline is broken, healing is slowed. Hopefully, the clinician can intervene when the timeline is broken and institute measures to promote completion of the healing process.

EXAM QUESTIONS

CHAPTER 2
Questions 8-14

8. An example of primary wound closure is

    a. healing of a pressure ulcer.

    b. immediate closure of a surgical incision.

    c. healing of a vascular ulcer.

    d. use of a skin graft.

9. With primary wound closure, epithelialization takes place in

    a. 24–36 hours.

    b. 7 days.

    c. 48–72 hours.

    d. 5 days.

10. The cells that are key in the wound healing process for partial-thickness wounds are

    a. fibroblasts.

    b. monocytes.

    c. myofibroblasts.

    d. epithelial cells.

11. Full-thickness wounds heal by

    a. scar formation.

    b. epithelial resurfacing only.

    c. surgical repair only.

    d. contraction and remodeling.

12. The main reparative function of the proliferative phase of wound healing is

    a. start of the wound healing cascade.

    b. deposition of connective tissue.

    c. vasodilation.

    d. degradation and resynthesis of collagen.

13. The wound healing phase that is characterized by edema, erythema, and tenderness of local tissues is

    a. inflammatory.

    b. proliferative.

    c. differentiation.

    d. primary.

14. The percentage of prewound tensile strength that scar tissue can obtain is

    a. 100%.

    b. 80%.

    c. 60%.

    d. 50%.

CHAPTER 3

FACTORS AFFECTING WOUND HEALING

CHAPTER OBJECTIVE

Upon completion of the chapter, the reader will be able to understand the systemic and local factors that can impact wound healing and recognize measures that can reduce factors that impede wound repair.

LEARNING OBJECTIVES

After completion of the chapter, the reader will be able to

1. list three local factors that can impede wound healing.

2. state five systemic factors that can impede wound healing.

3. explain the relationship between the wound healing process and factors that affect this process.

4. state three measures that can be taken to improve any detrimental wound repair effect from local and systemic influences.

INTRODUCTION

The information that was discussed in chapter 2 regarding the physiology of wound healing details a process that is complex yet well designed so that the majority of wounds that an individual can develop will repair in a satisfactory manner. It would be ideal if wound healing neatly followed the healing trajectory for all wounds, but that is not the case. Several factors can impede the healing process. Understanding how these factors affect wound healing can help the clinician choose treatment options that maximize the potential for desired outcomes and offer the individual the chance for wound repair that has an anatomic and functional result.

FACTORS THAT CAN IMPEDE WOUND HEALING

Wound repair is a systemic process that is affected by the host's overall condition. A variety of factors can interfere with and delay wound healing. Many of these factors are related to systemic disease processes. However, local factors at the wound site can also affect the healing process. Local factors include pressure, a dry wound environment, trauma, edema, infection, necrosis, foreign bodies, and incontinence. Systemic factors include age, body build, tissue oxygenation, chronic disease, nutritional status, vascular insufficiency, smoking, immunosuppression, and radiation therapy.

Local Factors

Pressure: If pressure is allowed to be applied in too great a force or for too long a period of time, that pressure can impede the blood supply to the wounded area, leading to delayed healing and possibly worsening the original wound.

Dry Wound Environment: Studies show that a moist would environment allows healing to occur three to five times faster than if the wound is allowed to dry out. Dry wound beds expose nerve endings, leading to increased pain and cell death. When wounds dry out and become desiccated, the cells of wound healing have a harder time migrating and performing their functions. Maintaining the goal of moist wound healing enhances cell migration and encourages epithelialization.

Trauma: A wound has a decreased chance of healing or possibly no chance at all if it continues to experience trauma. Therefore, wounds should be protected as much as possible from injury.

Edema: The presence of edema in the wound prevents the wound from obtaining the nutrients it needs to heal. Edema reduces the blood supply to the area and interferes with the transportation of oxygen and other nutrients needed for cellular function.

Infection: Any infection in the wound, either local or systemic, needs to be addressed in order for wound healing to progress. The cardinal signs of infection — induration, fever, erythema, and edema — need to be monitored, and if any of these signs occur, the physician needs to be contacted for appropriate treatment. Be aware of the chance of a silent infection or osteomyelitis in patients with chronic wounds with bone exposed or in wounds that do not appear to be responding to treatment. Abnormal wound cultures should be evaluated by the physician for appropriate treatment.

Necrosis or Foreign Bodies: Any foreign bodies in the wound bed, such as tubes, drains, or suture material, can impede the healing process. Necrotic tissue is also a deterrent to healing and an avenue for infection. Necrosis tends to be one of two main types: slough and eschar. Slough is usually yellow, hydrated, loose, and stringy; eschar is dehydrated, thick, black or brown, and leathery. Necrotic tissue and foreign bodies both impede wound repair and, therefore, need to be removed from the wound in order for healing to continue at an optimal rate.

Incontinence: Incontinence, whether urinary or fecal, can alter the integrity of the skin. Contamination or continued irritation by urine or feces makes it difficult for wound healing to proceed in an orderly fashion. Incontinence also makes care of the wound more difficult for the caregiver or clinician. Providing excellent incontinence management is essential for wound repair to continue unimpeded (Hess, 2002).

Systemic Factors

Age: With advancing age, multiple factors come into play with regard to wound healing. These factors include poor nutrition, dehydration, chronic diseases, poor mobility, vascular compromise, immunosuppression, and incontinence. The combination of these factors places an individual at an increased risk for skin breakdown and delayed wound healing. The clinician must perform comprehensive assessments in the aging population, including assessment of all of the factors that can affect the wound repair process.

Body Build: Initially, body build may not seem to have a significant impact on wound healing, however, when the clinician realizes that the vascular system is paramount in transferring oxygen and nutrients to the wound site, body build becomes important. In an obese individual, decreased blood supply to adipose tissue leads to decreased oxygen and nutrient distribution to the area. An emaciated individual has a similar problem — no nutritional stores to assist with wound healing (Hess, 2002).

Tissue Oxygenation: Tissue oxygenation and perfusion are essential for wound repair and healing. Oxygen is one of the main fuels for cellular function, and the amount of oxygenated blood at the wound site directly affects the repair process. Collagen synthesis and fibroblast differentiation both require oxygen for completion. The cells assisting in management of infection, such as the neutrophils and the macrophages, also depend on oxygen for their infection-fighting capabilities. Transcutaneous oxygen tension is the actual measurement of the oxygen on the skin surface. Levels that are considered to represent reasonable circulation to allow wound healing and to fight infection range from 30-40 mmHg. Chronic disease states that interfere with adequate tissue oxygenation and perfusion need to be addressed by the clinician. Disease states such as hypotension, trauma, sepsis, hypovolemia, and cardiac impairment may lead to hypoxia. Disease states that interfere with the capillary basement membrane, such as diabetic angiopathy, peripheral vascular disease, and radiation exposure, also restrict tissue perfusion and need to be addressed (Bryant, 2000; Makelbust & Sieggreen, 2001).

Chronic Disease: Chronic disease states can greatly affect wound healing either by involvement of the medication needed for the disease or by the comorbid conditions that go along with the disease. Side effects of medications, such as corticosteroids, can inhibit epithelial proliferation as well as the inflammatory phase of wound healing. Inhibition of the inflammatory response can be extremely detrimental. Delayed migration of neutrophils and macrophages into the wound increases the risk of infection and delays the healing cascade of events. The knowledge that vitamin A therapy can partially counteract the effects of steroids can assist the clinician in treatment measures (Bryant, 2000). Diabetes mellitus is one of the chronic disease states that greatly affects wound healing. High blood glucose values compete with cellular transport of ascorbic acid, which is essential for the deposition of collagen. Studies have also shown reduced ten-

sile strength and decreased connective tissue in patients with diabetes. Another effect of diabetes is the development of peripheral neuropathy. The presence of a neuropathic limb often results in the occurrence of a traumatic wound without the patient's knowledge. If the patient gets wounded, the inflammatory response is diminished secondary to leukocyte malfunction and the risk of infection becomes a problem. The comorbid condition of occlusive arterial disease also complicates healing because diminished blood flow to the wound means that oxygen and nutrients cannot reach the area (Bryant, 2000; Maklebust & Sieggreen, 2001).

Nutritional Status: Recognition of the importance of nutrition in wound healing has grown over the last several years. It is now an integral part of wound care management. When the initial wound assessment is done, a thorough nutritional assessment should be obtained as well, including the patient's use of vitamin and mineral supplements. Laboratory values that can be utilized to evaluate nutritional status include serum albumin, pre-albumin, and total protein. A dietitian should be consulted in order to obtain the appropriate information on nutrients and calories that are required for each patient's wound repair. Here is a list of some of the necessary nutrients, their importance, and their affect on wound repair.

Vitamin A: for collagen synthesis and epithelialization; deficiency leads to poor wound healing.

Vitamin C: for membrane integrity; deficiency leads to scurvy, poor wound healing, and capillary fragility.

Vitamin K: for coagulation; deficiency leads to increased risk of hemorrhage and hematoma formation.

Pyridoxine, Riboflavin, and Thiamine: for antibody and white blood count (WBC) formation, cofactors in cellular development, and enzyme activity facilitation; deficiency leads to decreased resistance to infection.

Copper: for collagen cross-linking; deficiency leads to decreased collagen synthesis.

Iron: for collagen synthesis and enhanced leukocyte bacterial activity; deficiency leads to anemia, which can result in increased risk of local tissue ischemia; impaired tensile strength of tissues; and impaired collagen cross-linking.

Zinc: for cell proliferation and cofactor for enzymes; deficiency leads to impaired healing, alteration in taste, and anorexia.

Proteins: for wound repair, clotting factor production, white blood cell (WBC) production and migration, cell-mediated phagocytosis, fibroblastic proliferation, neovascularization, collagen synthesis, epithelial cell proliferation, wound remodeling; deficiency leads to poor wound healing, edema, lymphopenia, and impaired cellular immunity.

Albumin: for control of osmotic equilibrium; deficiency leads to hypoalbuminemia, which promotes generalized edema and therefore slows oxygen diffusion and metabolic transport from the capillaries and cell membranes.

Carbohydrates: for the supply of cellular energy and protein sparing; deficiency leads to expenditure of visceral and muscle proteins for energy.

Fats: for the supply of cellular energy, the supply of essential fatty acids, cell membrane manufacture, and prostaglandin production; deficiency impedes tissue repair.

Arginine: for assistance in local wound immune system (has a high concentration of nitrogen, used in wound healing, and is the precursor to proline, which is converted to hydroxyproline and then to collagen). Deficiencies of arginine, an amino acid of protein, will have the same effects as protein deficiency.

Glutamine: for primary fuel for fibroblasts; helps to preserve lean body mass. Implications of deficiencies are unknown.

Vascular Insufficiency: The importance of the vascular system to wound repair and resolution has already been mentioned. Vascular compromise in the lower extremities can lead to arterial, venous, and pressure ulcers. If tissues do not receive the oxygen and nutrients they need, they cannot perform their vital functions. If a limb is suspected of vascular insufficiency, a suggestion for referral should be made to the physician to see if revascularization or medication is appropriate (Hess, 2002).

Smoking: The nicotine from smoking reduces vascular blood flow in two ways: 1) it is a potent vasoconstrictor and 2) it increases platelet adhesiveness, leading to clot formation. Cigarette smoke is also a vasoconstrictor and the carbon monoxide in it interferes with the oxygen carrying capacity of hemoglobin. It may also cause changes in the endothelium of the blood vessels and increase platelet adhesion, thereby limiting blood flow. Finally, the hydrogen cyanide in cigarette smoke inhibits the enzymes needed for oxygen transport and oxidative metabolism. Individuals who smoke and are anticipating surgery for pressure ulcer repair need to understand the increased risk of graft failure and should be encouraged to stop smoking (Maklebust & Sieggreen, 2001).

Immunosuppression and Radiation Therapy: Diseases or medications that suppress the immune system can impede wound healing and resolution mainly by reducing the inflammatory response and the healing cascade. This leads to an increased risk of infection. Radiation therapy many times changes or damages underlying tissues, leading to problems with the body's ability to effectively move oxygen and nutrients to the area (Hess, 2002).

SUMMARY

Many factors can affect how well wound healing progresses along the healing trajectory. In planning a treatment regimen for a patient or evaluating the effectiveness of a treatment, the clinician should consider local factors such as pressure, wound environment, trauma, edema, infection, necrosis, or foreign body involvement. Systemic factors can also affect healing, so the patient's age, body build, chronic disease states, nutritional status, vascular status, and immunological status must be accounted for in the wound healing equation. The basic needs must be met, such as tissue oxygenation and adequate blood flow, in order to obtain the outcome of wound repair. Efforts at promoting factors that encourage wound repair and eliminating or downgrading factors that have a negative impact should make a difference in the wound healing outcome.

EXAM QUESTIONS

CHAPTER 3
Questions 15-20

15. One local factor that affects wound healing is

    a. edema.

    b. age.

    c. body build.

    d. nutritional status.

16. The treatment that would help counteract local deterrents to healing is

    a. vitamin A therapy.

    b. additional protein snacks.

    c. control of diabetes mellitus.

    d. removal of necrotic debris in the wound.

17. The factor that may be present in a patient with poorly controlled diabetes that would alter wound healing rate is

    a. low glucose levels.

    b. decreased deposition of collagen.

    c. increased tensile strength.

    d. corticosteroid effects.

18. The portion of wound resolution and repair that vitamin K is important to is

    a. collagen synthesis.

    b. connective tissue synthesis.

    c. coagulation.

    d. WBC formation.

19. The portion of wound repair that vitamin A is important to is

    a. WBC formation.

    b. collagen synthesis and epithelialization.

    c. collagen synthesis alone.

    d. bone marrow proliferation.

20. One systemic factor that affects wound healing is

    a. dry environment.

    b. trauma and edema.

    c. immunosuppression.

    d. pressure.

CHAPTER 4

WOUND ASSESSMENT AND DOCUMENTATION

CHAPTER OBJECTIVE

Upon completion of the chapter, the reader will be able to state the importance of accurate and timely wound assessment and documentation. The reader will also be able to discuss parameters routinely used for wound assessment and documentation and how these factors can be evaluated to assess overall wound repair.

LEARNING OBJECTIVES

After completion of the chapter, the reader will be able to

1. state the reasoning behind accurate and timely wound assessment and documentation.

2. indicate three ways to classify wounds.

3. relate three options for measuring wounds.

4. describe five parameters used in wound assessment.

INTRODUCTION

Wound assessment and documentation is a critical component in the overall wound management plan. Without accurate and timely assessment, the clinician is unable to evaluate wound repair or degeneration that has occurred during the treatment plan. Assessments drive treatment decisions concerning the frequency of care, type of dressing, and use of other adjunctive therapies for wound healing. Unfortunately, wound assessment and documentation are not always completed or, if completed, are not always done with consistency or reliability. Often, different instruments are used in wound assessment or measurement and different reviewers provide differing opinions on wound progression. These difficulties have led to inabilities to effectively evaluate wound treatments and outcomes, yet the need for a consistent method of measurement still remains a goal (Bryant, 2000).

ANATOMY OF THE WOUND

The introduction to this chapter relates the importance of accurate assessment and documentation as critical components of wound management. The remainder of the chapter describes the assessment parameters used most often in this evaluation process. How do we use these parameters to know if the wound is healing or degenerating? Wound evaluation actually is quite complex and sometimes difficult to capture. The healing process, as well as the many different types of wounds, makes it difficult to evaluate all of the assessment parameters using one tool. The available tools look at prediction of wound development, current classification of a wound, measurement of a wound, and assessment of wound status that describes essential wound characteristics (Bryant, 2000).

A simplistic form of wound evaluation is that the clinician notices improvement in the wound. Wound repair is usually taking place when the following set of factors is present

- The overall size of the wound is smaller.*

- The depth of the wound is diminishing.*

- The drainage is decreasing in amount.*

- The tissue in the wound bed is showing less necrosis, if present, and more of a beefy red color as the wound fills in with granulation tissue.

- No foul odor is present in the wound or the drainage. The wound should be cleansed prior to the assessment of odor. Many dressings have odor upon removal due to their occlusive nature; this will be discussed in more detail in Chapter 9.

- The drainage is thinning and becoming a serosanguineous color.

- New epithelium appears on the wound margins.

- The wound margins are not macerated, thick, and rolled.

- The skin surrounding the wound is intact and is not inflamed or indurated.

- Tunneling and undermining are either absent or decreasing in size.

Patient assessment should be performed when the wound is initially being assessed and periodically during the management of the wound. Some of the patient assessment components in the history should include

- etiology, such as from trauma, pressure, or diabetes

- treatments that have been attempted in the past and their success rates

- wound duration (acute or chronic)

- oxygen saturation levels

- age

- additional systemic factors, such as disease processes the patient has that could affect wound healing

- use of medications, such as prednisone or nonsteroidal anti-inflammatory drugs

- recent laboratory values

- environmental factors, such as use of a wheelchair or cushions, and ambulation patterns.

A psychosocial assessment is also helpful when managing the patient with a wound. Some of the psychosocial aspects to investigate include

- depression

- social support and caregiver availability

- mental status

- barriers to learning and learning styles

- alcohol and drug use

- smoking history

- sexuality

- goals, lifestyle, and values

- stressors

- polypharmacy

- culture and ethnicity.

(Milne, Corbett, & Dubuc, 2003)

WOUND ASSESSMENT AND DOCUMENTATION PARAMETERS

Several physical parameters are evaluated when assessing wound status. The use of all of these parameters on a consistent basis allows the clinician to judge the repair process so that any necessary change in treatment can be instituted. The following parameters are used most frequently in assessment

1. Anatomical location

2. Wounds classification

   a. Staging, depth, or grade of wound

   b. Partial- versus full-thickness

   c. Color

---

*A wound may show signs of improvement but actually increase in size, depth, and drainage. When a large amount of necrotic tissue is liquefying as a result of autolysis or enzymatic debridement, the wound may measure larger and deeper with an increase in exudate. This is often confusing to clinicians who are not familiar with this process. It is also an important concept to communicate to caregivers and family members.

3. Wound measurement

4. Presence of undermining or tunneling

5. Type of tissue in wound bed

6. Exudate

7. Surrounding skin/wound margins

8. Duration of the wound

9. Pain with wound care or in the wound in general

Anatomical Location

The anatomical location can give an indication of the etiology of the wound. If the wound is located over a bony prominence, the etiology will often be pressure related. If the wound is located on the lower leg, not necessarily over a bony prominence, the wound is a vascular or neuropathic ulcer. Understanding the etiology of the wound helps the clinician evaluate and select the appropriate treatment modalities and healing potential. A second reason for stating the anatomical location is that it helps a second clinician know if new wounds develop that were not previously noted. This helps in the evaluation of the current treatment regimen (Bryant, 2000; Hess, 2002).

Wound Classification

Wounds are classified by either describing the level of damaged tissue observed or the color of the tissue visualized at the wound base.

Staging — Staging wounds looks at the wound in terms of tissue layers. The system used most often by the National Pressure Ulcer Advisory Panel consists of four basic stages:

Stage I: An observable pressure-related alteration of intact skin, which when compared to adjacent skin or the opposite area of the body, reveals changes in one or more of the following conditions: skin temperature (warmth or coolness), tissue consistency (firm or boggy), or sensation (pain or itching). The ulcer presents as a defined area of persistent redness in patients with lightly pigmented skin; in patients with darker skin tones, it may appear as persistent red, blue, or purplish hues.

Stage II: Partial-thickness skin loss involving the epidermis or dermis, or both. The ulcer is superficial and presents clinically as an abrasion, blister, or shallow crater.

Stage III: Full-thickness skin loss involving damage or necrosis of subcutaneous tissue, which may extend down to, but not through, the underlying fascia. The ulcer presents clinically as a deep crater with or without undermining of adjacent tissue.

Stage IV: Full-thickness skin loss with extensive destruction, tissue necrosis, or damage to muscle, bone, or supporting structures, such as a tendon or joint capsule.

A few limitations of the staging system need to be noted

a. A clinician cannot stage a wound that is covered with necrotic tissue until the base of the wound can be visualized. The documentation for this wound would be stated as "Unable to stage wound secondary to dry, black eschar." (See Figure 4-1.)

b. It may be difficult to accurately stage wounds in darkly pigmented skin.

c. The staging system was set up to evaluate pressure ulcers.

The staging system is constantly being reevaluated to improve the reliability and validity of the tool (Maklebust & Sieggreen, 2001).

Partial- versus full-thickness — These terms are used to describe the extent of tissue damage.

Partial-thickness – Skin damage is confined to the skin layers and does not penetrate through the dermis. The damage may only involve the epidermis. These wounds tend to heal by epithelialization only.

Full-thickness – Skin damage extends below the dermis into the subcutaneous layer and may also involve the muscle and supporting structures. Full-thickness wounds tend to heal by neovascularization, fibroplasia, and contraction (Bryant, 2000).

Color — The color system is a method of evaluating the wound based on the observed tissue. The three color classifications are black, yellow, and red.

Black – The wound is covered with necrotic tissue or eschar (dry, black-brown, leathery, nonviable tissue). (See Figure 4-1.) Eschar often covers an underlying necrotic process and is many times mistaken for a scab.

Yellow – The wound is various shades of yellow, from pale ivory to yellow-grey (slough tissue=necrotic debris). (See Figure 4-2.) Yellow wounds actively generate wound fluid.

Red – The wound has a pale pink to beefy red wound base. The beefy red wound bed indicates healthy granulation tissue. (See Figure 4-3.) (Bryant, 2000)

FIGURE 4-1
Unstageable Wound

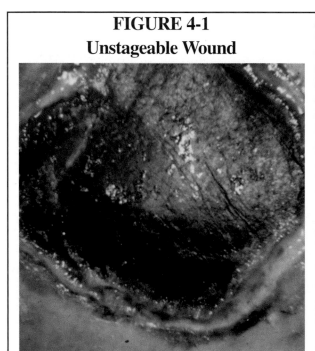

Unable to stage wound secondary to dry, black eschar.

FIGURE 4-2
Yellow, Stringy Slough Tissue

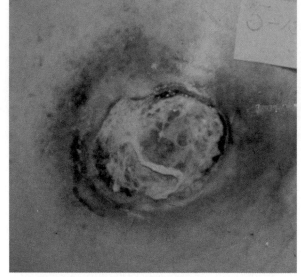

FIGURE 4-3
Granulation

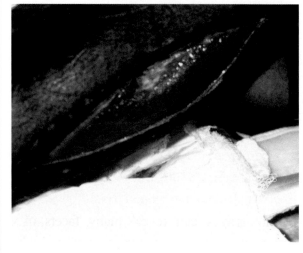

Beefy red granulation tissue over 90–95% of the wound, status post fasciotomy for compartment syndrome.

Wound Measurement

Wound measurement is one of the fundamental parameters that is used to judge healing and resolution of a wound. Wounds can be evaluated in either a two- or three-dimensional measurement. *Two-dimensional* measurements include linear measurement, wound tracings, and wound photographs. *Three-dimensional* measurements include linear measurements, wound molds, foam dressings, and fluid instillation.

Two-Dimensional Measurements

1. **Two-dimensional linear measurements** look at length and width of a wound but do not look at depth. This method is one of the simplest and most inexpensive ways to evaluate a wound. Linear measurements should be done in centimeters, not inches, and should be performed in a consistent manner to increase the reliability and validity of the readings. Various disposable plastic and paper measuring devices are available. The actual steps in linear measurement are discussed in the three-dimensional measurement section because that type of measurement is done most often.

2. In **wound tracings,** the external surface or perimeter of the wound is traced using transparent paper and a marking pen. These tracings can be done in a serial manner, offering pictures of either wound progression or deterioration. The surface area of a wound can also be calculated with wound tracings. Several commercial wound tracing products are available. The use of a two-piece tracing method can assist in avoiding contamination of the medical record.

3. **Wound photographs** are often used in conjunction with some other form of measurement. Photographs can reveal many facets of the wound and serial pictures can convey the healing or deterioration process. All photographs require consent from the patient. Any health care facility or agency practicing wound photography should have a written protocol regarding this practice. Photography is an art, and a variety of cameras and other equipment are available for wound assessment. Due to the variability in wound photographs, the expense that is incurred with photography, and the legal issues surrounding photography, not all health care facilities and agencies use this method of

documentation. The main issue is that the clinician must follow the protocol that has been established by the facility with respect to documenting with photography (Bryant, 2000).

Three-Dimensional Measurements

1. **Linear measurements,** as described above, are the easiest and most cost-effective method of wound measurement. Three-dimensional linear measurements, which look at length, width, and depth, are used most often. In taking these measurements, the wound should be envisioned as a clock, with the patient's head being at 12 o'clock and the patient's feet at 6 o'clock. The length readings should be obtained by aligning the measurement guide by the wound and reading the measurements from the long axis of the body. The width measurement is obtained by looking at the horizontal axis of the body. Three o'clock is at the patient's left side, and 9 o'clock is at the patient's right side. The depth of the wound is gauged by placing a cotton-tipped applicator into the deepest area of the wound and then holding the applicator with a gloved finger at the area where it becomes flush with the skin. The cotton-tipped applicator is then removed from the wound and held in place with the gloved finger, marking where the applicator became flush with the skin, along the measuring guide to obtain a reading. The complete three-dimensional linear reading should be recorded as length × width × depth and, once again, the reading should be in centimeters for uniformity.

2. **Wound molds** are another method of measuring the volume of open wounds. In this procedure, an alginate mold (see chapter 9) is used to fill the wound opening. As the liquid thickens, the mold can be removed and weighed for fluid volume displacement. With serial molds, the volumes displaced can be evaluated for wound repair. This method is not used often secondary to time, cost, and storage.

3. **Foam dressings** work in a similar fashion as alginate molds for measuring wound volume, however, they are made of a silicone elastomer product. This method of measurement is not utilized in the United States on a regular basis.

4. **Fluid instillation** evaluates fluid volume in the open wound. This procedure calls for the installation of either sterile normal saline solution or sterile water into the wound and then withdrawal of the instilled fluid via a syringe. The withdrawn volume is then measured. Serial recordings once again can lead to an indication of wound healing and repair. Some difficulties can arise with this method of wound measurement depending upon patient positioning and the possibility of fluid retention within the wound, which can lead to incorrect readings (Bryant, 2000).

Whichever method of wound measurement is utilized by the health care facility or agency, clinicians need to apply as much accuracy and precision as possible in obtaining the readings and must strive for consistency with each reading. This is important because all the tools that are currently used have validity and reliability issues.

Presence of Undermining or Tunneling

In assessing full-thickness wounds, other assessment parameters to look for are tunneling and undermining. Tunneling tends to be used to describe a narrow passage within the wound, whereas undermining is more of a larger lip or sweeping space under the wound margins. Tunneling and undermining can give the clinician an idea of how well the wound is progressing overall. It is once again important to be precise when measuring for tunneling and undermining. To measure for these assessment parameters, look at the patient as a clock, with the head at 12 o'clock and the feet at 6 o'clock, and then measure the tunneling or undermining in relation to the patient's positioning. Place a cotton-tipped applicator into the wound and gently probe until the end of the tunnel has been located. Place a gloved finger on

the cotton-tipped applicator at the point where the applicator is flush with the skin and then measure this area in centimeters. Two centimeters of tunneling at the top margin of a midabdominal wound would be described as "2 cm of tunneling at 12 o'clock." For undermining, the clinician would probably have a larger area to measure, but the measurements are taken in the same manner. An example of documenting undermining in the same abdominal wound described in the previous example would be: "3 cm of undermining from 12–2 o'clock and 6 cm of undermining from 6–9 o'clock." As with all measurements, accuracy and consistency are of utmost importance.

Type of Tissue in the Wound Bed

Describing the type of tissue in the wound bed also relays a good amount of information concerning the status of the wound and what treatments can be instituted. The tissue may range from viable (with a pale pink to beefy red granulation base), to nonviable (with a tan, yellow, brown, or black base). Stating whether the tissue is granulation tissue versus tendon, muscle, or another supporting structure adds to the description of the wound. Using a percentage to clarify your description of the wound bed is also helpful (for example, "The wound bed is 50% beefy red granulation tissue and 50% yellow, stringy slough tissue"). Always evaluate the wound bed for foreign bodies, such as suture material or other surgical material that could affect wound healing (Bryant, 2000).

Exudate

Exudate should be evaluated for many characteristics including amount, color, odor, and consistency. The amount of exudate can be described as a percentage of the dressings that is being saturated or by the frequency of dressing changes. A description of the color should also be stated (for example, serosanguineous, bloody, tan, light green, or yellow). Odor can be described as foul or malodorous or absent. Finally, the consistency of the exudate should be described as thin, watery, or creamy. The characteristics of the exudate let the clinician know if the wound is progressing normally or if complications, such as infection, are present (Bryant, 2000).

Surrounding Skin and Wound Margin

Wound margins or edges can let the clinician know if healing is progressing. New epithelium on the edges indicates progress toward wound resolution. Conversely, thick, white, rolled edges indicate a chronic condition where little improvement is taking place. Absence of epithelial tissue is an indication that treatment needs to be adjusted.

The condition of the surrounding skin is also an excellent indicator of whether the current treatment regimen is working. Is the surrounding skin red, warm, or indurated. Does it show signs of infection? Is the skin macerated or dry and flaking (indicates the level of moisture retention)? Are papules, pustules, vesicles, rashes, ecchymotic areas, or other discolorations present? These assessments provide a wealth of information on the status of the wound and the general condition of the patient, which in turn guides the clinician in the institution of correct treatment modalities (Bryant, 2000).

Duration of the Wound

The duration of the wound provides an idea of where on the healing trajectory the wound should be. If the patient has a new surgical wound, the clinician can expect a healing ridge after about 7 days. An incision or acute wound that is not following the healing trajectory needs intervention. A chronic pressure or vascular ulcer also needs some form of intervention if the wound is not following some type of healing or resolution within a selected time frame. The treatment plan should be evaluated every 2–3 weeks for any needed adjustments (Bryant, 2000).

Pain Associated with the Wound

Pain associated with a wound may be related to the wound itself or to the type of dressing that is being used. Removal of the dressing at the dressing change can also cause pain. Wound pain can be debilitating, affecting the patient's quality of life and general well-being. Pain is a subjective measure and there are a variety of pain scales that the clinician can utilize to document the patient's pain associated with a wound. The pain scales should be used on a routine basis to assist the clinician in evaluating the treatment plan and what deciding measures should be instituted.

Some general principles can help guide the clinician's in management of wound pain. The clinician should assess all patients for wound pain, eliminate or control the source of the pain, and provide analgesia as needed and appropriate. The clinician should evaluate the wound for infection, because infection can cause pain at the wound site. Moist wound healing principles should also be used with the dressing change so that the wound bed is disrupted as little as possible. Additional topical treatments can be instituted to spare the periwound skin from damage. Clinicians can also reduce wound care pain by having a gentle hand when changing the dressings. These measures should help the patient with a wound obtain a more comfortable level during the wound repair phase (Krasner & Kane, 2001).

DOCUMENTATION

Many different tools are available for wound assessment and documentation, and any one alone may not obtain the desired information for specific assessment situations. The clinician may need to utilize a combination of tools and documentation methods to reach the desired outcome. A few of the more well-known wound assessment scales or tools for healing include: 1) Pressure Sore Status Tool (PSST), 2) Sessing Scale, 3) Pressure Ulcer Scale for Healing (PUSH), 4) Wound Healing Scale, and 5) Sussman Wound Healing Tool (SWHT) (Milne, Corbett, & Dubuc, 2003). Photographic documentation can be used to supplement these wound healing tools and is usually discussed in the health care agency's policy and procedure guidelines. Photographic documentation of the wound is taken upon admission; whenever the wound changes, at predetermined, selected intervals; and upon discharge. The legal implications associated with photo documentation must be considered by the facility administrators when deciding the facility's policy regarding the use of photos (Hess, 2002).

Assessment and documentation schedules are usually set by the policy of a health care facility or agency. In the acute setting, wound assessment may be necessary on a daily basis or with each dressing change; whereas in the long-term care or home health setting, wound assessment 1 to 2 times a week may be sufficient. The goal for wound assessment and documentation is that it be done at the frequency dictated and that it is as precise as possible, allowing for the best information to be obtained in order to evaluate the stated outcomes (see Figure 4-4). Documentation should be a picture of what the clinician sees. Based on the wound documentation, colleagues should be able to get an excellent picture in their minds of what the wound looked like, and they should be able to evaluate the treatment regimen for any needed adjustments in therapy.

SUMMARY

The importance of wound assessment and documentation cannot be overstated. Accurate and frequent assessments guide the wound management team in making appropriate decisions for wound care. The documentation that results from the use of specified parameters should give a picture of what the clinician sees when evaluating the wound. The parameters that are most frequently used in the assessment process include anatomical location, wound measurement in three-dimensional linear measurements, presence of undermining or tunneling, type of tissue in the wound bed, type and amount of exudate, condition of the surrounding skin and wound margins, duration of the wound, and pain associated with the wound or with the dressing change. The wound is also classified by either the staging method, the color method, or the extent of tissue damaged, such as partial- or full-thickness involvement. When wound assessment and documentation is done in a consistent manner using specified parameters, treatments can be evaluated for their efficacy and adjustments or adjunctive therapies can be instituted to achieve the desired outcomes.

FIGURE 4-4
WOUND ASSESSMENT AND DOCUMENTATION PROGRESS REPORT

Write in the appropriate code to describe the wound characteristic.

Anatomical Location	Wound Type	Size	Undermining (clock method)	Wound Color	Amount	Drainage Color	Odor	Surrounding Skin

Pressure Ulcer Stage: _____

WOUND DESCRIPTIVE CODES
(Use as many as appropriate.)

Wound Type
V = Venous
A = Arterial
N = Neuropathic
I = Incision
D = Denuded
B = Burn
S = Skin tear
O = Other
P = Pressure

Wound Color
(Use %)
R = Red
Y = Yellow
Bl = Black
P = Pink
W = White
T = Tan
O = Other

Drainage Amount
(Saturation of drsg.)
N = None
Sc = Scant < 25%
Sm = Small 25%
M = Mod. 50%
L = Large 75%
Sat = Saturated 100%

Drainage Color
S = Serous
SS = Serosang
Y = Yellow
T = Tan
G = Green
B = Brown

Drainage Odor
N = None
M = Mild
S = Strong
F = Foul
O = Other

Surrounding Skin
I = Intact   ID = Indurated
D = Dry   C = Callous
F = Flaking   B = Bruising
M = Macerated   S = Scarring
E = Erythema

Specialty Bed:_____

Current Wound Care and Comments:_____

_____

_____

Nurse's Signature:_____Date: _____

Patient Name:_____MR #:_____

EXAM QUESTIONS

CHAPTER 4
Questions 21-29

21. The staging system classifies wounds based on

    a. surface area of involved tissue.

    b. tissue layers that are involved.

    c. color of the involved tissue.

    d. condition of the surrounding skin.

22. An ulcer that is superficial and presents as an abrasion, blister, or shallow crater should be classified as

    a. Stage I.

    b. Stage II.

    c. Stage III.

    d. Stage IV.

23. The three colors that are used in the color classification system are

    a. tan, green, and red.

    b. tan, yellow, and red.

    c. black, yellow, and red.

    d. brown, black, and yellow.

24. With regard to wound photography, which statement is true?

    a. Photographs should be taken of all patient wounds for documentation.

    b. Consent is needed before a photograph is taken.

    c. Photographs must be taken by a 35-mm camera.

    d. Photographs can stand alone as acceptable wound documentation.

25. Accurate and timely wound assessments are valuable for the clinician because they

    a. comply with regulations.

    b. are for documenting only.

    c. keep the patient aware of progress.

    d. evaluate current treatment and allow adjustment of therapy as necessary.

26. Three-dimensional linear measurements should be documented as

    a. width × length × depth.

    b. length × width × depth.

    c. depth × length × width.

    d. depth × width × length.

27. When describing undermining or tunneling of a wound using the clock method, the area of tunneling in the direction of the patient's feet would be

    a. 8 o'clock.

    b. 6 o'clock.

    c. 3 o'clock.

    d. 12 o'clock.

28. The presence of an epithelial margin indicates

    a. the treatment should be adjusted because no healing is occurring.

    b. evidence of infection.

    c. evidence of healing and wound improvement.

    d. maceration of the surrounding skin.

29. The parameters used most frequently in wound assessment are

    a. anatomical location, size, exudate, wound base and margins, and surrounding skin.

    b. anatomical location, wound margins, and surrounding skin.

    c. size, exudate, wound base and margins, and surrounding skin.

    d. size, exudate, and wound base and margins.

CHAPTER 5

MANAGEMENT OF ACUTE SURGICAL WOUNDS

CHAPTER OBJECTIVE

Upon completion of the chapter, the reader will be able to identify the acute surgical wound, and factors that affect wound healing, explain care of the incision, recognize abnormalities in the healing process, and understand when to follow up with the physician. The reader will also be able to present the options for caring for surgical donor sites and basic information on care of surgical flaps and grafts.

LEARNING OBJECTIVES

After completion of the chapter, the reader will be able to

1. state four factors affecting healing of acute wounds.

2. discuss appropriate treatment for an incision.

3. recognize the sequence of healing events for an acute wound.

4. list three local changes at the incision site that should be monitored.

5. identify two options for treating surgical donor sites.

INTRODUCTION

The definition of an acute wound was introduced in chapter 2, where wound healing was discussed. As stated in that chapter, the acute surgical wound usually heals rapidly without any complica-tions and follows the healing trajectory. Although acute surgical wounds heal uneventfully in most cases, the healing process is still quite complex and is affected by multiple factors that can lead to complications. These complications can lead to the need for additional surgical interventions that require the wound care clinician to understand the basic care of surgical flaps, grafts, and donor sites.

THE ACUTE SURGICAL WOUND

The acute surgical wound is one that has been closed by primary intention, or primary closure; as a result, the tissue defect and the risk of infection are minimized. The amount of connective tissue or scar tissue that is required to repair the defect is much smaller than that required for a wound healing by secondary intention. Acute surgical wounds still proceed through the repair process of inflammation, angiogenesis, fibroplasia, matrix deposition, and epithelialization, but this process is less noticeable to the clinician. Furthermore, the repair process is much faster with the surgical incision. Since the repair process is faster, the clinician needs to perform accurate assessments to be sure that healing is progressing appropriately (Bryant, 2000).

FACTORS AFFECTING THE HEALING OF ACUTE SURGICAL WOUNDS

Once again, there are many factors that can affect the healing rate and complications associated with incisional closure. A few of the indirect factors that affect acute wound healing include the type of preoperative and perioperative protocols in place with regard to infection control, the methods of skin prepping prior to surgery, types of suture materials used, and the length of hospitalization before surgery was completed.

Direct factors associated with the patient's systemic condition, such as chronic disease states, malignancy, nutritional status, circulation, blood oxygen concentration, and the methods of caring for the wound, also affect wound healing. As previously mentioned, the clinician can focus on these factors to optimize wound healing conditions and to institute protocols to assist with wound healing rates (Bryant, 2000).

Incision Care

The first postoperative dressing is many times referred to as the primary dressing and has the functions of protecting the new incision, absorbing drainage, and maintaining a sterile environment. Absorptive, nonadhesive dressings are a good choice postoperatively for preventing rewounding of the incision with the dressing change. If drainage is present, gauze dressings commonly stick to the incision as the drainage is wicked up into the gauze fibers. Incisions are usually kept clean and dry with no routine cleansing protocol unless soiled. Reepithelialization of the wound is usually completed 2–3 days after surgery. At this point, in theory, the wound is closed to bacterial contamination and no longer requires a dressing. However, the wound still does not have tensile strength and is subject to trauma so the patient and physician may prefer to leave a dressing in place a few days longer for protection (Bryant, 2000).

The usual closure materials include metal staples or clips, sutures, and steri-strips. Steri-strips provide an alternative to the microwounds (small openings in the skin along the margins of the main incision) that are created when metal staples or clips or suture materials are used. A problem arises with steri-strips when there is too much drainage that loosens the adhesive and compromises wound closure. On the other hand, staples and sutures that have been left in place too long, have been pulled too tight, or have become taut with tissue edema can lead to increased inflammation and potential infection and complications. The clinician needs to keep abreast of the time elapsed since surgery and when the closure materials should come out. Depending on the surgical procedure, metal clips or sutures are usually replaced by steri-strips in 1–2 weeks (Bryant, 2000).

CHANGES AT THE INCISION SITE

One of the most important indicators of wound progression is the healing ridge. This ridge results from the deposition of collagen, which begins in the inflammatory phase and peaks in the proliferative phase of wound healing. This accumulation of collagen can be felt as a ridge or induration of tissue, usually extending approximately 1 cm on either side of the incision during days 5–9 after surgery. Concern arises when no ridge is felt, because this may lead to dehiscence and infection often accompanies dehiscence. Additional changes at the wound site include discoloration, induration, increased temperature or pain at the incision site, or drainage coming from a previously dry and intact wound. These changes can signify an infection or hematoma and the surgeon should be notified immediately. If the incision does open and continues to have drainage, local wound care is usually performed until the wound heals by secondary intention (Bryant, 2000).

COMPLICATIONS WITH INCISION HEALING

Wound Dehiscence

Wound dehiscence has been defined as "separation of the layers of a surgical wound; it may be partial and superficial only, or complete with disruption of all layers" (Dorland's Illustrated Medical Dictionary, 2003) (see Figure 5-1). Dehiscence usually takes place early on in the postoperative period, when the healing ridge is being laid down and the tensile strength is low. At this time, the tissues are vulnerable to stresses, such as abdominal distention, ileus, or respiratory difficulties. Factors affecting wound healing, such as age, nutritional status, chronic disease states, and vascular insufficiency, can also lead to wound dehiscence. The release of collagenase at the wound margins during the normal healing process (part of collagen deposition and

FIGURE 5-1
Dehisced Surgical Wound

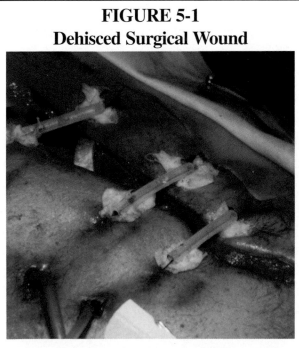

ICU patient with abdominal dehiscence. Note strips of Vaseline® gauze around retention sutures to minimize erosion.

remodeling) can also lead to incision breakdown. If the patient is compromised, the collagenase may weaken the tissues surrounding the sutures or clips, leading to tissue failure. Incision dehiscence may require immediate surgery to repair the defect and prevent possible evisceration. If the defect does not present any immediate danger, local wound care utilizing the principles of moist wound healing may be instituted until the wound heals by secondary intention (Carabasi & Jarrell, 1991).

Scar Formation

Scar formation varies from one individual to another. The remodeling of scar tissue and collagen deposition continue for 1–2 years, so the cosmetic appearance of the scar may change as time passes. A hypertrophic scar is composed of dense fibrous tissue that results from excessive collagen synthesis. The scar appears as a tense, reddish tissue ridge and is usually accompanied by itching, hyperesthesia, and tenderness. Etiology of the scar is unknown. These scars are most commonly seen in dark-skinned patients as well as younger patients. There are two types of hypertrophic scars: ordinary hypertophic scar and keloid.

Ordinary hypertrophic scar: This scar histologically shows an increased amount of normal collagen and a large number of mature fibroblasts with a small amount of ground substance. The scar is within the confines of the wound and usually stabilizes in about 3 months and may even regress and soften.

Keloid: This scar histologically shows large, swollen eosinophilic collagen bundles with a large amount of ground substance and scant fibroblasts. Keloid tissues invade nearby normal tissue that was not part of the original wounding. Keloid tissues tend to enlarge even after about 6 months and show no signs of regression or softening.

Treatment for hypertrophic scarring is difficult because excision of the scar may lead to a recurrence. Radiation therapy or steroid injections into the scar may prevent recurrence. Silicone dressings have been used in treating scar formation, and carbon dioxide laser treatment has also shown positive results (Carabasi & Jarrell, 1991; Maklebust & Sieggreen, 2001).

BASIC WOUND MANAGEMENT FOR SURGICAL GRAFTS AND FLAPS

At times, the management of a surgical wound involves the use of a flap or graft in the final closure.

Postoperative care of a split-thickness skin graft includes:

1) Protecting the area from trauma.

2) Protecting the area from outside contaminants.

3) Insulating the graft site.

4) Absorbing excessive exudate.

Usually, a bulky compression dressing and possibly a splint are used postoperatively. The surgeon usually removes the first dressing to evaluate the site and provides the instructions for care and a time when the splint is to be removed. The initial dressing may stay in place 5 to 7 days after surgery. The immobilization period depends on the graft site, surgery, and surgeon's preference.

Postoperative care of a myocutaneous flap includes:

1) Protecting the operative sites from trauma.

2) Keeping the suture line clean and dry.

3) Eliminating pressure over the flap site, drain sites, donor sites, and suture lines.

4) Protecting the surgical site from contaminants, such as incontinence.

5) Keeping the drains patent and functioning.

Postoperative care of the flap site also involves monitoring for signs and symptoms of infection or seroma. The initial dressing is changed by the surgeon, who instructs the clinician on the desired dressing change and frequency of change. Drains are commonly left in for up to 5 days and then removed when the amount of drainage has decreased. Measures to decrease pressure, friction, and shearing must be instituted. The patient is usually supported by some form of pressure-relieving surface to manage these factors. Sutures are usually left in place for up to 21 days (Krasner & Kane, 2001).

MANAGEMENT OF SURGICAL DONOR SITES

The donor site, also known as the graft harvest site, is a fast-healing wound. However, it is an acute wound that must be addressed to reduce the risk of external contamination and wound infection. Factors that affect the healing rate of the donor site include the site, size, and depth of tissue removed. The donor site for burns many times is a partial-thickness wound that heals by re-epithelialization. In the management of burns, one donor site may be harvested several times during the course of grafting, but the healing may be prolonged with evidence of hypertrophic scarring. The donor site for pressure ulcers or other full-thickness wounds may involve incisions that require care until they close by primary intention (Bryant, 2000; Young & Fowler, 1998).

Important considerations with donor site management include external contamination, infection, and pain. Pain may be the primary concern, and the patient may complain of more pain from the donor site than from the grafted area. This is especially true if the donor site involves a split-thickness depth where the nerve endings are left exposed. An ideal donor site dressing is one that is easy to apply, minimizes leakage of wound fluid, promotes re-epithelialization, and decreases the patient's pain. Older methods of managing donor sites have included tulle gras, low-adhering dressings, and leaving the donor site open to air. However, these methods cause considerable pain. With the advent of newer wound care products, a variety of options are available to decrease donor site pain and promote healing. Some of these options include calcium alginates, semipermeable films, xeroform gauze, hydrocolloids, and silicone-based dressings. All of these products reduce pain during donor site management (Young & Fowler, 1998).

DOCUMENTATION FOR ACUTE SURGICAL WOUNDS

Documentation of how the incision or surgical wound looks is extremely important in discovering problems in the wound healing process. The earlier a problem can be identified, the quicker the intervention can be instituted for improved wound healing. Accurate documentation with wound healing is also needed to maintain the patient's record for facility and legal purposes. It is difficult to remember what a wound or incision looked like weeks or months ago if it was not documented. Accurate documentation also drives the decision-making process regarding the type of wound management that is used. Without proper documentation, the clinician has inadequate input to make effective decisions on the plan of treatment. Complete documentation is essential for appropriate care of the surgical patient (Moore & Foster, 1998).

Detriments to accurate documentation include lack of time, low staff-to-patient ratio, and increased primary care or hands-on time required for the patient. These factors all limit the time for documentation. Even though these detriments are present, tools exist to assist in the standardization of acute surgical incision and wound documentation. These assessment tools need to be both valid and reliable in order to provide optimal outcomes. Two

types of tools that can effectively be used to document incision and wound healing include wound healing charts and wound care pathways.

Documentation for incision healing must include many factors, such as the location of the incision, number of days since surgery, size of the incision or wound, presence of any remaining closure materials, color of the incision, presence or absence of epithelial resurfacing, presence or absence of the healing ridge, type and amount of exudate, type of dressing used, and any action or referral. These parameters can be captured on the wound healing tool, graph, chart, or pathway, but the parameters should be captured consistently with each surgical incision or wound evaluation (Sussman & Bates-Jensen, 2004).

SUMMARY

Knowing the factors that affect incision healing, understanding the normal wound healing phases, and recognizing changes at the wound site should give the clinician the assessment skills necessary to recognize deviations and potential problems in healing of the acute surgical wound. This information should also arm the clinician with methods to optimize healing, to institute appropriate protocols, and to notify the physician of complications so that a positive outcome is achieved. When closure of the surgical wound requires a flap or graft, understanding the basic management of these wounds and donor site care can assist the clinician in obtaining improved healing while promoting patient comfort and satisfaction.

EXAM QUESTIONS

CHAPTER 5
Questions 30-36

30. The clinician's role in the success of primary closure of the acute surgical wound is

    a. following preoperative and perioperative protocols with regard to infection control.

    b. choosing the type of suture material used.

    c. giving the patient a good breakfast the morning of surgery.

    d. communicating to the family during the operative procedure.

31. An appropriate dressing choice for a new postoperative incision would be

    a. hydrocolloid dressings.

    b. gauze dressings.

    c. absorbent, nonadhesive dressings.

    d. hydrogel dressings.

32. Depending on the surgery, staples or sutures are usually removed postoperatively after

    a. 3–5 days.

    b. 5–7 days.

    c. 7–14 days.

    d. 21 days.

33. The healing ridge of the incision is usually present postoperatively by

    a. 1–3 days.

    b. 3–5 days.

    c. 5–9 days.

    d. 10 days.

34. A postoperative incision complication that can occur when the healing ridge is compromised and the tensile strength is low is known as

    a. infection.

    b. dehiscence.

    c. induration.

    d. irritation.

35. Two good options for the treatment of surgical donor sites include

    a. calcium alginate dressings and xeroform gauze.

    b. hydrocolloid dressings and normal saline dressings.

    c. calcium alginate dressings and hydrogel dressings.

    d. leaving the donor site open to air or covering it with a dry dressing.

36. Four factors that affect healing of the acute wound include

    a. nutritional status, circulation, preoperative protocols, and type of suture materials.

    b. chronic disease states, nutritional status, infection control methods, and socioeconomic factors.

    c. circulation, blood oxygen concentration, socioeconomic factors, and perioperative protocols.

    d. chronic disease states, infection control methods, circulation, and family environment.

CHAPTER 6

RISK ASSESSMENT AND PRESSURE ULCER PREVENTION

CHAPTER OBJECTIVE

Upon completion of the chapter, the reader will have a greater understanding of the factors that place a patient at risk for skin breakdown and pressure ulcer formation. The reader will also be familiar with risk assessment tools and how to use them. The reader will recognize measures to institute to prevent the occurrence of skin breakdown.

LEARNING OBJECTIVES

After completion of the chapter, the reader will be able to

1. report five factors that place the patient at risk for skin breakdown and pressure ulcer formation.

2. identify the uses of a risk assessment tool.

3. discuss how malnutrition affects tissue integrity.

4. list five ways of positioning a patient in bed to decrease pressure.

5. state five ways of positioning a seated patient to decrease pressure.

6. demonstrate the use of support surfaces with pressure ulcer prevention methods.

7. relate four ways to promote intact skin and prevent pressure, friction, and shearing.

8. identify three goals for patient and family education regarding pressure ulcer prevention.

INTRODUCTION

The prediction and prevention of pressure ulcers has been studied quite extensively in the last several years. As a result, excellent guidelines have been developed as standards to assist clinicians with their practice. Screening tools have been created to identify patients at greatest risk for pressure ulcers, and a set of protocols has been instituted to help reduce, if not prevent, debilitating ulcers. Factors that are targeted in the prevention of pressure ulcers include nutritional status, mechanical loading, support surfaces, and skin care. The Agency For Healthcare Research and Quality (formerly known as the Agency For Health Care Policy and Research [AHCPR]) has made available patient and clinician pressure ulcer prevention guidelines. These guidelines are now used as the standard of care and should be a part of every clinician's practice. The "Pressure Ulcer Prediction and Prevention Algorithm" from the *AHCPR Clinical Practice Guidelines: Pressure Ulcers in Adults: Prediction and Prevention* displays the management paths that are undertaken to predict and prevent pressure ulcers and offers areas to investigate for specific interventions to the risks that are identified (see Figure 6-1).

RISK ASSESSMENT

Assessing for pressure ulcer risk is based on the knowledge that soft tissue breaks down more easily under certain conditions and that there are several intrinsic patient conditions or factors that lead to pressure ulceration. Listed here are several variables that are associated with pressure ulcer development

*   chronological age

*   number and type of medical diagnoses

*   mental status/level of consciousness

*   nutritional status

*   immobility/ability to move independently

*   chronicity of health problems

*   incontinence/bladder and bowel control

*   adequacy of circulation

*   presence of infection or fever.

The higher the number of risk factors or variables a patient has, the higher the chance of pressure ulceration. Certain patient populations tend to be high-risk groups. Quadriplegics are one such population group. Another patient population at risk are intensive care unit patients. One study found a 60% pressure ulcer prevalence rate in quadriplegics and a 33% pressure ulcer prevalence rate for intensive care unit patients (Bryant, 1992).

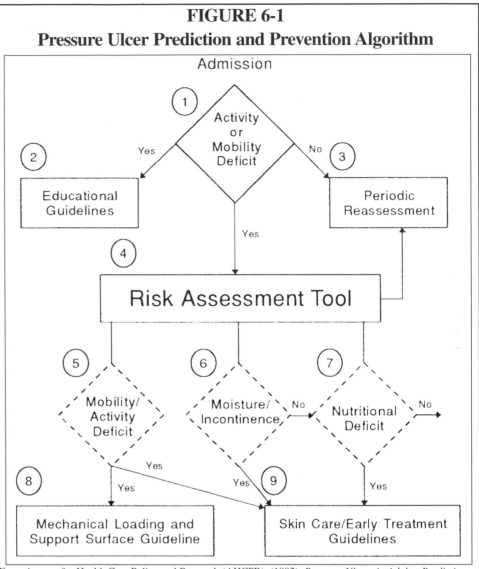

FIGURE 6-1
Pressure Ulcer Prediction and Prevention Algorithm

From Agency for Health Care Policy and Research (AHCPR). (1992). *Pressure Ulcers in Adults: Prediction and Prevention. Clinical Practice Guideline* Number 3, Pub. No. 92-0047. National Library of Medicine. Retrieved April 6, 2004 from http://hstat.nim.nih.gov/

RISK ASSESSMENT TOOLS

The occurrence of pressure ulcers is an extremely costly consequence, not only in terms of dollars utilized for care but also for the debilitating effects on the patient and family. Fortunately for both the health care industry and the patient, several tools have been developed to identify individuals at risk for pressure ulcer development. These screening tools vary from inexpensive rating scales to serum albumin testing, to more sophisticated laser Doppler flow studies. These tools differ in their invasiveness, cost, reliability, and validity. The tools that have been shown to provide the highest reliability and validity are the rating scales; these tools also happen to be the least invasive and least costly. The two main rating scales that are used are the Norton scale and the Braden scale (Braden & Bergstrom, 1996).

Norton Scale

The Norton scale consists of five parameters that look at physical condition, mental condition, activity, mobility, and incontinence. Each parameter has four descriptors that are rated from 4 to 1. The descriptors for each parameter are listed below.

	4	3	2	1
Physical Condition	Good	Fair	Poor	Very Bad
Mental Condition	Alert	Apathetic	Confused	Stupor
Activity	Ambulant	Walk/help	Chairbound	Bed
Mobility	Full	Slightly limited	Very limited	Immobile
Incontinence	None	Occasional	Usually/ Urine	Doubly

A patient is evaluated on the above parameters and then given a total score. The total score can range from 5–20, with lower scores indicating a higher risk for pressure ulcer formation. Norton found that there was an almost linear relationship between the scores of elderly patients and the formation of pressure ulcers. A score of 14 indicated "onset of risk," and a score of 12 or below indicated high risk for incidence of pressure ulcers. Consult one of the wound care texts listed in the reference section for a full description and copy of the Norton scale (Bryant, 1992).

Braden Scale

The Braden scale consists of six subscales that reflect sensory perception, skin moisture, activity, mobility, nutritional intake, and friction and shear (see Figure 6-2). Sensory perception rates how well the patient responds to pressure-related discomfort. Skin moisture rates the degree to which skin is exposed to moisture. Activity rates the patient's overall degree of physical activity. Nutrition rates the patient's usual food pattern. Friction and shear rate how much force the skin takes with movement. The subscales are rated from 1–4, except friction and shear, which is rated from 1–3. The total scores can range from 6–23. The lower the score, the lower the functional level and the higher the risk for pressure ulcer formation (Braden & Bergstrom, 1996). A stable adult patient with a score of 16 or below is considered at risk. For elderly patients, a score of 17–18 may be a more correct predictor of pressure ulcer incidence secondary to comorbid factors (Bryant, 1992).

Research using these rating scales has found them to be extremely predictive of pressure ulcer formation. Some studies have shown that 95–100% of patients who scored an 11 or less on the Braden scale went on to develop a pressure ulcer. All of the full-thickness ulcers that developed were observed in patients classified in the highest risk category. A risk assessment tool is the backbone of a pressure ulcer prevention program and, with its utilization, not only is the incidence of pressure ulcers decreased but the cost associated with the prevention program is decreased as well (Braden & Bergstrom, 1996).

WHO SHOULD ASSESS RISK?

Risk assessment and pressure ulcer prevention practices are performed routinely by many health care team members, but who should perform the rating scales? The rating scales need to have reliability and validity with each measurement. Extensive studies show that the best results with validity and reliability were assessments by registered nurses. There are a few options to improve the reliability and validity scores: the registered nurse can consult directly with the staff involved in the completion of the rating scale or the facility may

FIGURE 6-2

PRESSURE ULCERS IN ADULTS — CLINICAL PRACTICE GUIDELINE

BRADEN SCALE — For Predicting Pressure Sore Risk

HIGH RISK: Total score ≤12
MODERATE RISK: Total score 13-14
LOW RISK: Total score 15-16 if under 75 years old OR 15-18 if over 75 years old.

RISK FACTOR	SCORE/DESCRIPTION				DATE OF ASSESS. →		
					1	2	3	4
Sensory perception Ability to respond meaningfully to pressure-related discomfort	**1. Completely limited:** Unresponsive (does not moan, flinch, or grasp) to painful stimuli, due to diminished level of consciousness or sedation. OR limited ability to feel pain over most of body surface.	**2. Very limited:** Responds only to painful stimuli. Cannot communicate discomfort except by moaning or restlessness. OR has a sensory impairment which limits the ability to feel pain or discomfort over 1/2 of body.	**3. Slightly limited:** Responds to verbal commands but cannot always communicate discomfort or need to be turned. OR has some sensory impairment which limits ability to feel pain or discomfort in 1 or 2 extremities.	**4. No impairment:** Responds to verbal commands. Has no sensory deficit which would limit ability to feel or voice pain or discomfort.			
Moisture Degree to which skin is exposed to moisture	**1. Constantly moist:** Skin is kept moist almost constantly by perspiration, urine, etc. Dampness is detected every time patient is moved or turned.	**2. Moist:** Skin is often but not always moist. Linen must be changed at least once a shift.	**3. Occasionally moist:** Skin is occasionally moist, requiring an extra linen change approximately once a day.	**4. Rarely moist:** Skin is usually dry, linen requires changing only at routine intervals.			
Activity Degree of physical activity	**1. Bedfast:** Confined to bed.	**2. Chairfast:** Ability to walk severely limited or nonexistent. Cannot bear own weight and/or must be assisted into chair or wheelchair.	**3. Walks occasionally:** Walks occasionally during day but for very short distances, with or without assistance. Spends majority of each shift in bed or chair.	**4. Walks frequently:** Walks outside the room at least twice a day and inside room at least once every 2 hours during waking hours.			
Mobility Ability to change and control body position	**1. Completely immobile:** Does not make even slight changes in body or extremity position without assistance.	**2. Very limited:** Makes occasional slight changes in body or extremity position but unable to make frequent or significant changes independently.	**3. Slightly limited:** Makes frequent though slight changes in body or extremity position independently.	**4. No limitations:** Makes major and frequent changes in position without assistance.			
Nutrition Usual food intake pattern	**1. Very poor:** Never eats a complete meal. Rarely eats more than 1/3 of any food offered. Eats 2 servings or less of protein (meat or dairy products) per day. Takes fluids poorly. Does not take a liquid dietary supplement. OR is NPO[1] and/or maintained on clear liquids or IV[2] for more than 5 days.	**2. Probably inadequate:** Rarely eats a complete meal and generally eats only about 1/2 of any food offered. Protein intake includes only 3 servings of meat or dairy products per day. Occasionally will take a dietary supplement. OR receives less than optimum amount of liquid diet or tube feeding.	**3. Adequate:** Eats over half of most meals. Eats a total of 4 servings of protein (meat, dairy products) each day. Occasionally will refuse a meal, but will usually take a supplement if offered. OR is on a tube feeding or TPN[3] regimen, which probably meets most of nutritional needs.	**4. Excellent:** Eats most of every meal. Never refuses a meal. Usually eats a total of 4 or more servings of meat and dairy products. Occasionally eats between meals. Does not require supplementation.			
Friction and shear	**1. Problem:** Requires moderate to maximum assistance in moving. Complete lifting without sliding against sheets is impossible. Frequently slides down in bed or chair, requiring frequent repositioning with maximum assistance. Spasticity, contractures, or agitation leads to almost constant friction.	**2. Potential problem:** Moves feebly or requires minimum assistance. During a move skin probably slides to some extent against sheets, chair, restraints, or other devices. Maintains relatively good position in chair or bed most of the time but occasionally slides down.	**3. No apparent problem:** Moves in bed and in chair independently and has sufficient muscle strength to lift up completely during move. Maintains good position in bed or chair at all times.				

Total score of 12 or less represents HIGH RISK

TOTAL SCORE		EVALUATOR SIGNATURE/TITLE	ASSESS.	DATE	EVALUATOR SIGNATURE/TITLE
ASSESS.	DATE				
1	/ /		3	/ /	
2	/ /		4	/ /	

NAME—Last, First, Middle

ATTENDING PHYSICIAN

ID NUMBER

[1]NPO: Nothing by mouth. [2]IV: Intravenously. [3]TPN: Total parenteral nutrition

desire to have a training session designed to instruct licensed vocational nurses and nursing assistants who conduct the rating scales and then offer sufficient practice and feedback to obtain more consistent rating scores (Braden & Bergstrom, 1996).

TIMING OF ASSESSMENTS

The timing of assessments depends upon the clinical setting. It is recommended for all settings that an initial assessment be performed on patient admission and again 24–48 hours later as well as whenever the patient's condition changes. Routine assessments every 24 hours after initial admission are recommended in intensive care units; in acute care units, every other day; in skilled nursing units, weekly for the first 4 weeks and then quarterly thereafter. Some skilled nursing facilities continue to perform monthly assessments. In home health care, frequency should be determined by the primary registered nurse case manager who is familiar with the client's status.

NUTRITION

The value of nutrition was already discussed in chapter 3 as a factor that affects wound healing. As such, it also can be presumed to be a factor in prevention. Nutrition is important in the maintenance of tissue integrity. The patient and family need to be instructed in this relationship for good nutritional management. Healthy adults need 0.8 gram of protein per kilogram of body weight and sufficient calories to maintain metabolic needs. If these needs are not met, the body breaks down glycogen and fat reserves, putting the body in a state of negative nitrogen balance and jeopardizing tissue integrity.

Laboratory tests and physical measurements can assist the clinician in evaluating a patient's nutritional status. Serum protein, serum albumin, transferrin, and pre-albumin levels are indicators of nutritional status. The longer a patient has been malnourished,

the lower the levels of these indicators. Normal levels for these tests are as follows:

Protein:	6.0–8.0 g/dl
Albumin:	3.5–5.0 g/dl
Transferrin:	200–400 mg/dl
Pre-albumin:	20–40 mg/dl

The formation of pressure ulcers has been associated with severely malnourished individuals. Hypoalbuminemia is considered severe when levels are < 2.5 g/dl. Patients in this state need alternative ways to obtain nutrition.

If a previous weight can be used for reference, body weight can also be an excellent predictor of nutrition problems. A nurse, dietitian, or physician should be notified of any unintentional weight loss of 10 pounds or greater during a 6-month period. For a patient at risk for malnutrition, a 5% change in body weight that is unintentional can be predictive of a drop in serum albumin. Understanding these relationships can help the clinician set nutritional goals with the patient and family. A patient may need supplemental feedings or vitamins and minerals in addition to regular methods of obtaining nutrition. A dietitian should be consulted for assistance with options for meeting the patient's dietary needs, especially if malnutrition is suspected. Dietitians have a wealth of knowledge and are an integral part of the wound care team. To evaluate the outcomes of the treatment regimen, patients who are at risk for malnutrition need to have their weights and laboratory values monitored regularly as well as have nutritional assessments done at least every 3 months (Maklebust & Sieggreen, 1996).

MECHANICAL LOADING

The goal with regard to mechanical loading and support surfaces is to protect the patient against the adverse effects of external mechanical forces: pressure, friction, and shear. A direct relationship exists between unrelieved pressure of a significant intensity and duration and the occurrence of tissue necrosis and ulceration; therefore, interrupting the intensity and duration can help to reduce the occurrence of pressure ulcers (see Figure 6-3).

FIGURE 6-3
Ischium

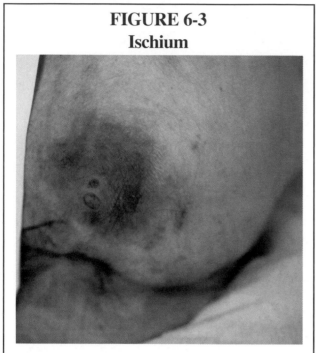

Small ischial full-thickness wound with peri-wound erythema. This is a sitting injury and pressure relief in the chair needs to be addressed.

Suggestions for positioning the patient's body in ways that will decrease or relieve pressure, friction, and shear are included in the following list.

Positioning while in bed

- Do not position the patient on a reddened area of the body.
- Do not use donut-shaped devices.
- Place the patient in a 30-degree, laterally inclined, side-lying position when turning, but never position the patient over the greater trochanter of the femur.
- Elevate any extremity that has a reddened area.
- Use pillows and foam wedges to keep bony prominences apart and protected.
- Suspend the patient's heels off of the mattress to relieve pressure; even if the patient is on a specialty bed.

- Keep the head of the patient's bed elevated less than 30 degrees, except for meals, or per the patient's tolerance, secondary to other medical complications.
- Turn the patient at least every 2 hours (more often if redness is present).
- Position pillows above the sacrum and coccyx area to avoid pressure in the high risk area when turning patients on their side.
- Lift the patient across a surface rather than dragging.
- Use pullsheets, side rails, and an overbed frame with trapeze as devices to help bedridden patients reposition.
- Use a turning clock or other turning schedule to help remind staff of the need to turn bedbound individuals.
- Use socks, long sleeves, or some type of thin film or hydrocolloid dressing over the patient's heels and elbows to assist in decreasing the effects of friction and shearing.
- Avoid hazards of immobility by rehabilitating the patient with physical therapy to the individual's maximum functional level (AHCPR, 1992; Maklebust & Sieggreen, 1996).

Positioning while sitting

- Emphasize good body posture and alignment.
- Do not allow the patient to sit directly over reddened areas.
- Do not allow the patient to sit on donut-shaped devices.
- Keep the tops of the patient's thighs horizontal, so that weight is evenly distributed to the backs of the thighs and no extra pressure is applied to the ischia.
- Keep the patient's knees separated to prevent pressure and irritation.
- Ensure that the patient who can reposition without assistance changes his or her position every 15 minutes. If able, the patient should learn to

do wheelchair pushups every 15 minutes to relieve pressure or, if safety permits, should learn to lean forward to reduce pressure.

- Assist the patient who cannot relieve pressure unaided back to bed after 1 hour of chair sitting (AHCPR, 1992; Maklebust & Sieggreen, 1996).

SUPPORT SURFACES

Patients who are at risk for pressure ulcer development have a variety of support surfaces available to them — not only for the bed but for the wheelchair as well. Pillows and low-density foam cushions were the mainstay of support devices several years ago, but today a variety of products are available that are even more effective at pressure reduction. This section briefly touches on the products that are available, but it is recommended that the clinician discuss products and their uses with either a company representative or a specialist in support and seating surfaces at the health care facility/agency.

Support surfaces can be classified by three main functions: 1) to prevent skin breakdown in people who are immobile; 2) to prevent additional skin breakdown; and 3) to promote healing in an individual who already has skin breakdown in multiple areas.

In choosing the type of support surface that a patient may need, it is important to understand the theory behind the use of support surfaces. Support surfaces were designed to reduce tissue interface pressures over bony prominences by maximizing surface contact and redistributing the weight of the body over a larger area. Tissue interface pressure is a measurement of the amount of pressure between the skin and a resting surface. The goal of a support surface is to bring tissue interface pressure near to or at capillary closing pressure. Capillary closing pressures, which range from 12–32 mm Hg, are the guidelines by which support surfaces are judged in their pressure reduction or pressure relief capability. When capillaries become closed off or occluded

due to pressure, tissue ischemia develops, leading to the formation of ulcerations. Support surfaces, therefore, help to decrease or redistribute that pressure for patients at risk for ulcers or for the treatment of existing ulcers (Bryant, 2000).

Types of Support Surfaces

Support surfaces can be categorized using several methods. Listed below are methods for categorizing specialty surfaces. (See Figure 6-4).

I. Management of Pressure
- Pressure Reduction
- Pressure Relief

II. Air or Fluid Support
- Dynamic
- Static

III. Type of Device
- Overlay
- Replacement Mattress
- Specialty Bed

The first category of support surfaces is concerned with the management of pressure. This category contains pressure reduction devices and pressure relief support surfaces. Pressure reduction devices lower interface pressures of standard hospital mattresses or chair seating cushions, but they do not consistently reduce pressure to less than the standard capillary closing pressures. Pressure relief support surfaces consistently reduce the interface pressure below the stated capillary closing pressures and thus offer a higher degree of therapy.

The second category of support surfaces is air or fluid support, which is divided into dynamic and static surfaces. A dynamic system usually utilizes electricity to alternate between inflation and deflation in a pad- or bubble-type surface that decreases interface pressures. An alternating air pressure pad is an example of this type of surface. Static devices, on the other hand, reduce pressure by spreading the load over a greater surface area. The inflation level is held constant and is maintained by the use of

54

Chapter 6–
Wound Management and Healing

FIGURE 6-4
Medicare Part B Coverage for Support Surfaces in the Home Health Setting

Professional Practice Fact Sheet   **MEDICARE PART B COVERAGE FOR SUPPORT SURFACES IN THE HOME HEALTH SETTING**

Introduction
This fact sheet addresses Medicare Part B support surface coverage criteria and reimbursement guidelines. These guidelines apply to patients who are eligible for home health care services, but do not apply to acute, longterm or hospice care.

Coverage Criteria

Group I	Group II	Group III
A patient would qualify if they meet either of the following scenarios:	A patient would qualify if they meet one of the following scenarios:	A patient would qualify only if all of the following criteria are met: - The patient has a Stage III or IV ulcer. - The patient is bedridden or chair bound as a result of severly limited mobility. - In the absence of an air-fluidized bed, the patient would require institutionalization. - The air-fluidized bed is ordered in writing by the patient's attending physician based upon a comprehensive assessment and evaluation.
Scenario 1: The patient is completely immobile.	Scenario 1: The patient has multiple Stage II ulcers located on the trunk and/or pelvis, and - a comprehensive ulcer treatment program, including the use of an appropriate Group I support surface, has been tried for at least one month. - The ulcers have worsened or remained the same.	- A comprehensive ulcer treatment program, including the use of an appropriate Group II support surface, has been tried for at least one month with worsening or no improvement to the ulcer. - A trained adult caregiver is available to assist the patient with activities of daily living, repositioning, dietary and fluid needs, prescribed treatments, and management and support of the air-fluidized bed system and its problems. - A physician directs the home treatment regimen on a monthly basis. - All other alternative equipment has been considered and ruled out.
Scenario 2: The patient has limited mobility or any stage ulcer on the trunk or pelvis and has at least one of the following: - impaired nutritional status - fecal or urinary incontinence - altered sensory perception - compromised circulatory status.	Scenario 2: The patient has: - large or multiple Stage III or IV ulcer(s) located on the trunk or pelvis	
	Scenario 3: - The patient has had a recent myocutaneous flap or skin graft on the trunk or pelvis (surgery within the past 60 days). - The patient has been on a Group II or III product prior to discharge from a hospital or skilled nursing facility. Note: Patient coverage under this scenario is limited to 60 days post-op.	An air-fluidized bed will be denied under any of the following circumstances: - Co-existing pulmonary disease - Wet soaks or moist dressings that are not protected with an impervious covering. - Caregiver is unwilling or unable to provide the type of care required on an air-fluidized bed. - Structure support is inadequate to support the weight of the air-fluidized bed. - The electrical system is insufficient for the aniticpated increase in consumption.

FIGURE 6-4 (continued)
Medicare Part B Coverage for Support Surfaces in the Home Health Setting

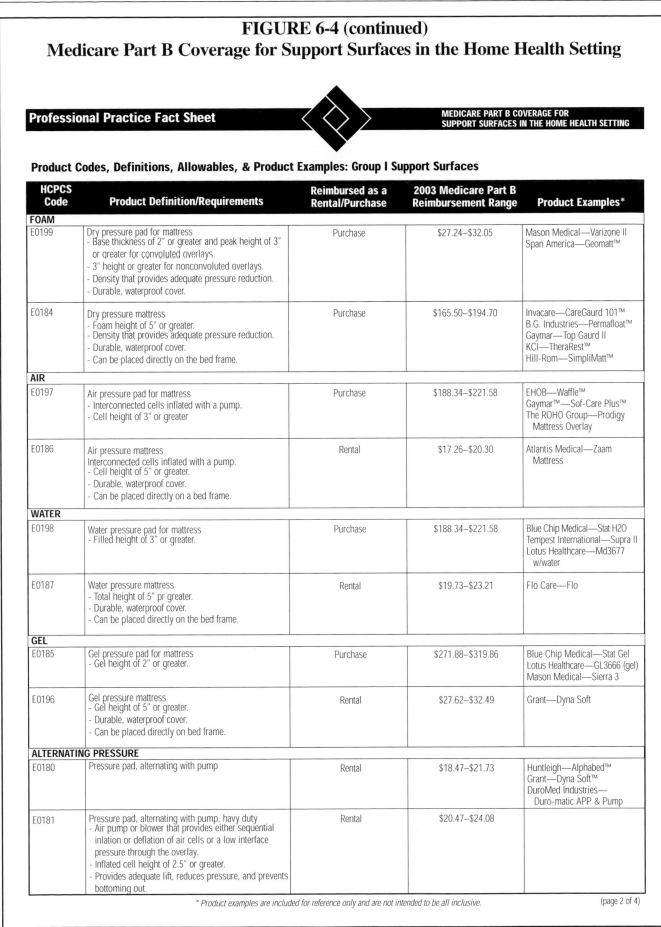

| **Professional Practice Fact Sheet** | ◆ | **MEDICARE PART B COVERAGE FOR SUPPORT SURFACES IN THE HOME HEALTH SETTING** |

Product Codes, Definitions, Allowables, & Product Examples: Group I Support Surfaces

HCPCS Code	Product Definition/Requirements	Reimbursed as a Rental/Purchase	2003 Medicare Part B Reimbursement Range	Product Examples*
FOAM				
E0199	Dry pressure pad for mattress - Base thickness of 2" or greater and peak height of 3" or greater for convoluted overlays. - 3" height or greater for nonconvoluted overlays. - Density that provides adequate pressure reduction. - Durable, waterproof cover.	Purchase	$27.24–$32.05	Mason Medical—Varizone II Span America—Geomatt™
E0184	Dry pressure mattress - Foam height of 5" or greater. - Density that provides adequate pressure reduction. - Durable, waterproof cover. - Can be placed directly on the bed frame.	Purchase	$165.50–$194.70	Invacare—CareGaurd 101™ B.G. Industries—Permafloat™ Gaymar—Top Gaurd II KCI—TheraRest™ Hill-Rom—SimpliMatt™
AIR				
E0197	Air pressure pad for mattress - Interconnected cells inflated with a pump. - Cell height of 3" or greater	Purchase	$188.34–$221.58	EHOB—Waffle™ Gaymar™—Sof-Care Plus™ The ROHO Group—Prodigy Mattress Overlay
E0186	Air pressure mattress Interconnected cells inflated with a pump. - Cell height of 5" or greater. - Durable, waterproof cover. - Can be placed directly on a bed frame.	Rental	$17.26–$20.30	Atlantis Medical—Zaam Mattress
WATER				
E0198	Water pressure pad for mattress - Filled height of 3" or greater.	Purchase	$188.34–$221.58	Blue Chip Medical—Stat H2O Tempest International—Supra II Lotus Healthcare—Md3677 w/water
E0187	Water pressure mattress - Total height of 5" pr greater. - Durable, waterproof cover. - Can be placed directly on the bed frame.	Rental	$19.73–$23.21	Flo Care—Flo
GEL				
E0185	Gel pressure pad for mattress - Gel height of 2" or greater.	Purchase	$271.88–$319.86	Blue Chip Medical—Stat Gel Lotus Healthcare—GL3666 (gel) Mason Medical—Sierra 3
E0196	Gel pressure mattress - Gel height of 5" or greater. - Durable, waterproof cover. - Can be placed directly on bed frame.	Rental	$27.62–$32.49	Grant—Dyna Soft
ALTERNATING PRESSURE				
E0180	Pressure pad, alternating with pump	Rental	$18.47–$21.73	Huntleigh—Alphabed™ Grant—Dyna Soft™ DuroMed Industries—Duro-matic APP & Pump
E0181	Pressure pad, alternating with pump, havy duty - Air pump or blower that provides either sequential inlation or deflation of air cells or a low interface pressure through the overlay. - Inflated cell height of 2.5" or greater. - Provides adequate lift, reduces pressure, and prevents bottoming out.	Rental	$20.47–$24.08	

* Product examples are included for reference only and are not intended to be all inclusive.

(page 2 of 4)

FIGURE 6-4 (continued)
Medicare Part B Coverage for Support Surfaces in the Home Health Setting

Professional Practice Fact Sheet

MEDICARE PART B COVERAGE FOR SUPPORT SURFACES IN THE HOME HEALTH SETTING

Product Codes, Definitions, Allowables, & Product Examples: Group II Support Surfaces

HCPCS Code	Product Definition/Requirements	Reimbursed as a Rental/Purchase	2003 Medicare Part B Reimbursement Range	Product Examples*
NONPOWERED				
E0371	Nonpowered, advanced pressure-reducing overlay - Height and design of individual cells provides significantly more pressure reduction than a Group 1 overlay. - Prevents bottoming out - Total height of 3" or greater. - Surface designed to reduce friction and shear. - Evidence that the product is effective in treating conditions described by Group II coverage criteria.	Rental	$377.81–-$444.48	ROHO—ROHO DRY FLOATATION™ Mattress System KCI—RIK Fluid Overlay™
E0373	Nonpowered, advanced pressure-reducing mattress - Height and design of individual cells provides significantly more pressure resuction than a Group I overlay. - Prevents bottoming out. - Total height of 5" or greater. - Surface designed to reduce friction and shear. - Evidence that the product is effective in treating conditions described by Group II coverage criteria. - Can be placed directly on a hospital bed frame.	Rental	$522.30–$614.47	KCI—RIK Fluid Mattress™ Span-America—Pressure Guard CFT™
POWERED				
E0372	Powered air overlay for mattress. - Air pump or blower which provides either sequential inflation and deflation or low interface pressure through the cells. - Inflated height of the air cells is 3.5" or greater. - Provides adequate lift, reduces pressure, and prevents bottoming out. - Surface that reduces friction and shear.	Rental	$458.44–$539.34	Plexus Medical—Air Express Hill-Rom—Acucair™ Huntleigh—Alpha Xcell KCI First Step Classic™
E0277	Alternating pressure mattress - Air pump or blower that provides either sequential inflation and deflation or low interface pressure through the cells. - Inflated height of the air cells is 5" or greater. - Provides adequate lift, reduces pressure, and prevents bottoming out. - Surface reduces friction and shear. - Can be placed directly on a bed frame,	Rental	$646.46–$759.36	Hill-Rom—Silkair™ KCI—First Step Tri-Cell™ Pegasus—Air Wave Therapeutic MRS™ Sen Tech Medical—Stage IV Invacare—MicroAir 3500S™ Huntleigh—DFS 2™ Air Care Therapy—Select Air
E0193	Powered air floatation bed - Semi-electric bed with a fully integrated powered pressure-reducing mattress. - Meets all of the requirements of E0277.	Rental	$767.94–$903.46	KCI—KinAir III

Product examples are included for reference only and are not intended to be all inclusive.

(page 3 of 4)

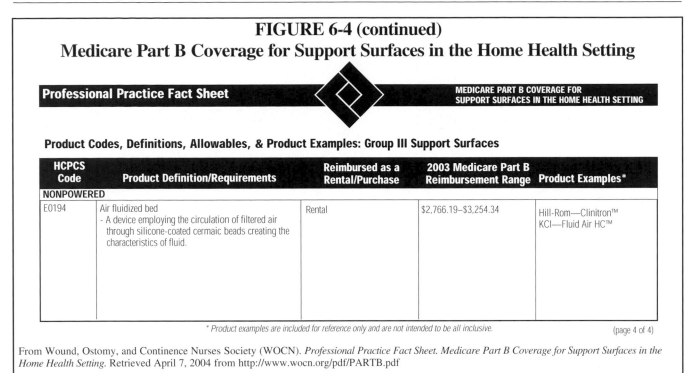

FIGURE 6-4 (continued)
Medicare Part B Coverage for Support Surfaces in the Home Health Setting

Professional Practice Fact Sheet

MEDICARE PART B COVERAGE FOR
SUPPORT SURFACES IN THE HOME HEALTH SETTING

Product Codes, Definitions, Allowables, & Product Examples: Group III Support Surfaces

HCPCS Code	Product Definition/Requirements	Reimbursed as a Rental/Purchase	2003 Medicare Part B Reimbursement Range	Product Examples*
NONPOWERED				
E0194	Air fluidized bed - A device employing the circulation of filtered air through silicone-coated cermaic beads creating the characteristics of fluid.	Rental	$2,766.19–$3,254.34	Hill-Rom—Clinitron™ KCI—Fluid Air HC™

* Product examples are included for reference only and are not intended to be all inclusive.

(page 4 of 4)

From Wound, Ostomy, and Continence Nurses Society (WOCN). *Professional Practice Fact Sheet. Medicare Part B Coverage for Support Surfaces in the Home Health Setting.* Retrieved April 7, 2004 from http://www.wocn.org/pdf/PARTB.pdf

materials that mold to the body surface, such as gel, water, foam and, occasionally, air-filled devices.

The third category is the type of device, such as an overlay, a replacement mattress, or a specialty bed. Overlay mattresses are applied on top of regular mattresses and utilize foam, air, water, or gel to redistribute the weight and reduce pressure. Replacement mattresses take the place of hospital mattresses and have built in foam or gel combinations that reduce pressure. These mattresses have been utilized more in the hospital setting as an alternative to overlays as a way to reduce costs. A specialty bed either replaces the standard hospital bed frame and mattress or is a special unit that replaces the mattress but can still be used on the hospital bed frame (Bryant, 2000).

The health care facility or agency usually has some type of algorithm or protocol in place to assist with decisions on when to place a patient on a specialty bed. These protocols usually consider mobility, respiratory status, incontinence, skin status, cost, environment, and long-term goals of therapy. It is suggested that each clinician become familiar with the health care facility's or agency's protocol before placing a patient on a support surface. Placing a patient on the incorrect support surface may not be beneficial to the patient and can be quite costly as well. The *AHCPR Clinical Guidelines: Treatment of Pressure Ulcers* include an algorithm for the management of tissue loads that is an excellent guide to begin with when evaluating a patient's needs. (See Figure 6-5.) (AHCPR, 1994)

It should be noted that egg crate mattresses are for comfort only, not pressure relief. The use of a therapeutic foam overlay as a pressure reducing device is recommended if it has these features

- base height of 3–4 inches.

- density of 1.3 to 1.6 pounds per cubic foot.

- 25% indentation load deflection (ILD) of about 30 lb.

All types of support surfaces have advantages and disadvantages. It is important in the decision-making process to weigh all of these factors against the patient's needs. In many cases, the guidelines for use are more restrictive or lenient than needed in the clinical setting. If the clinician is in a setting that allows for individualization, other factors should be considered. For example, a patient who has a full-thickness pressure ulcer on the sacrum qualifies per Medicare guidelines for low-air-loss therapy. This

FIGURE 6-5
Management of Tissue Loads

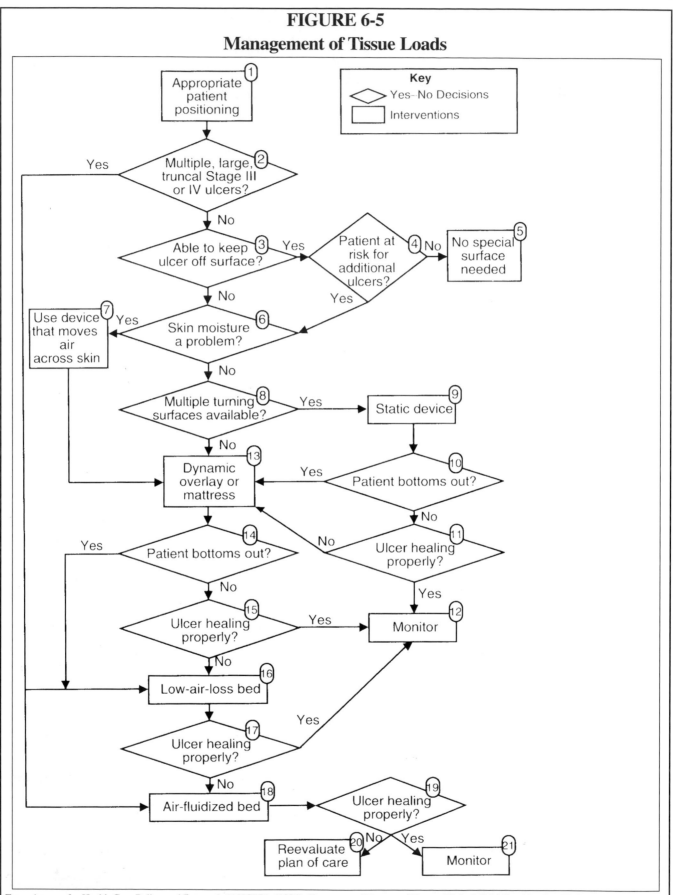

From Agency for Health Care Policy and Research (AHCPR). (1994). *Treatment of Pressure Ulcers*. Clinical Guideline Number 15, Pub. No. 95-0652. National Library of Medicine. Retrieved April 6, 2004 from http://hstat.nlm.nih.gov/

patient may be able to be positioned from side to side to avoid the area of the pressure ulcer. In this case, the clinician may choose to order a Group I product or a lower-priced Group II product, which could save a significant amount of money and still be adequate for the patient. Assessment and evaluation must be continual to ensure that wound progress is being made and, more importantly, that deterioration is not occurring. It is recommended that a clinician learn the generic categories of support surfaces and their specific characteristics in order to make informed decisions (Maklebust & Sieggreen, 2001). The choice of support surfaces is dynamic, and knowledge of products assists optimum choice for the patient.

Wheelchair Seating Considerations

Special wheelchair seating devices composed of foam, gel, air, or a combination of products are available. These products usually require measurements for a correct fit to the chair and the patient. There are special wheelchair seating clinics that patients can attend to be specially fitted for a cushion that will reduce pressure over the ischial tuberosities. Some of the factors that should be evaluated when considering a cushion are continence of bladder and bowel, cost, lifestyle, postural stability, and pressure evaluation (Maklebust & Sieggreen, 2001). Too often patients are placed on a therapeutic support surface for the bed and then sit up in a chair for hours without adequate support. It has been estimated that 75% of the sitting-dependent population will develop pressure ulcers and, of these, 75% will have a recurrence of the same breakdown (Sussman & Bates-Jensen, 2004). Correctly seating individuals in chairs is a critical component of healing and prevention of pressure ulcers. If wounds are on the ischium, they are pressure induced from sitting, and this area needs to be addressed. The other common sitting ulcer site is the sacrum. Although often attributed to shear and friction in the bed, sacral ulcers can also be caused by or at least enhanced by sitting in a chair. The way a person sits in a chair is just as important to assess

and treat as the body positioning in bed. Elderly patients typically slide down in their seats. Remember that no cushion on the market completely relieves all pressures; gravity is always at work. The goal is to distribute the weight more evenly across a surface to reduce the pressures over bony prominences. In addition, reinforcement of pressure-relieving measures while in the chair, as well as limited seating time, is of utmost importance.

SKIN CARE AND MANAGEMENT

A fourth area of concentration for pressure ulcer prevention is skin care. In the previous material on the anatomy and physiology of aging skin, comments were made concerning the ease of injury to the elderly population secondary to skin changes that have taken place. Decreased skin elasticity, decreased glandular secretions, increased dryness, and a thinner dermoepidermal junction were just a few of the reasons for problems with skin care and pressure ulceration formation. Healthy skin needs to be kept moisturized, soft, and supple. Both dry skin and excessively wet skin increase the risk of skin injury. Dry skin cracks, causing breaks in the skin. Heel fissures can develop from dryness, resulting in painful heels, and can progress to wounds. Excessively wet skin decreases the threshold of friction injury; therefore, caution should be used when lifting and transferring patients. The following interventions can be carried out to improve outcomes in the prevention of pressure ulcers with aged or at-risk skin:

- All patients at risk should have a systematic skin inspection at least once daily, paying particular attention to the bony prominences. The results of the skin inspection should be documented.

- Avoid massage over bony prominences.

- Minimize environmental factors that cause skin drying, such as low humidity (< than 40%) and exposure to cold.

- Treat dry skin with moisturizers.

- Cleanse the skin at the time of soiling and at routine intervals.

- Individualize skin cleansing according to patient preference and need.

- Use mild cleansing agents that minimize irritation, and avoid hot water.

- Use nonalkaline cleansing agents to preserve the acid mantle of the skin.

- Minimize force during cleansing to decrease the force and friction applied to the skin.

- Protect the skin from irritants, such as urine and feces, by using protective barrier ointments or incontinence collectors. Rectal tubes are not good alternatives for managing fecal incontinence because they may cause complications associated with vasovagal responses and ischemia of anal tissues.

- Use absorptive underpads to wick moisture away from the skin.

- Do not place plastic and paper linen pads next to the patient's skin, because they retain moisture.

- Diapers should only be used on patients when they are ambulating or up in a chair, not while lying in bed.

- As able, use lubricants, protective films, protective dressings, and protective padding to decrease the effects of friction and shearing.

- Use proper positioning, transferring, and turning techniques to decrease friction and shearing forces.

All interventions and outcomes should be monitored and documented so that the treatment plan can be adjusted as needed and so that continuity and consistency are met to obtain the best possible outcomes (AHCPR, 1992; Maklebust & Sieggreen, 2001).

EDUCATION

The goal of educational programs is to reduce the incidence of pressure ulcers by coordinated efforts on the part of the clinician, family, and patient. It has been suggested by the *AHCPR Clinical Practice Guidelines* that the educational program include the following information

- etiology and risk factors for pressure ulcers

- risk assessment tools and their application

- skin assessment

- selection and use of support surfaces

- development and implementation of an individualized program of skin care

- demonstration of positioning to decrease the risk of tissue breakdown

- instruction on accurate documentation of pertinent data.

(AHCPR, 1992).

SUMMARY

The fact that most pressure ulcers are preventable, coupled with the availability of information on prediction and prevention, would lead one to believe that the incidence and prevalence of pressure ulcers would be almost nonexistent; however, this is not the case. The presence and incidence of pressure ulcers, especially in certain populations, reinforces the need for continued diligence on the part of the clinician in educating the patient and family and in keeping abreast of the current trends in prevention and prediction techniques.

EXAM QUESTIONS

CHAPTER 6
Questions 37-51

37. The factors associated with pressure ulcer development are

    a. nutritional status, chronological age, and adequacy of circulation.

    b. nutritional status, chronological age, and socioeconomic status.

    c. financial status, chronological age, and adequacy of circulation.

    d. nutritional status, cultural orientation, and adequacy of circulation.

38. An example of a noninvasive risk screening tool for pressure ulcer prediction is the

    a. Glascow scale.

    b. Apache score.

    c. Wagner scale.

    d. Braden scale.

39. The five parameters of the Norton Scale include

    a. physical condition, friction, shearing, nutrition, and mentation.

    b. physical condition, mental state, activity, mobility, and incontinence.

    c. friction, shearing, nutrition, mobility, and incontinence.

    d. friction, nutrition, shearing, physical condition, and mobility.

40. The score that indicates "onset of risk" with the Norton Scale is

    a. 18.

    b. 16.

    c. 14.

    d. 12.

41. The Braden scale is composed of

    a. four subscales.

    b. five subscales.

    c. six subscales.

    d. seven subscales.

42. Risk assessment is recommended to be performed in an intensive care unit

    a. every 24 hours.

    b. every other day.

    c. every 12 hours.

    d. once a week.

43. Routine assessment is recommended to be performed in a home health setting

    a. only when the patient's status changes.

    b. every week.

    c. as ordered by the primary nurse.

    d. monthly.

44. To maintain normal metabolic needs, healthy adults need

    a. 0.6 gram of protein per kilogram of body weight.

    b. 0.8 gram of protein per kilogram of body weight.

    c. 1.0 gram of protein per kilogram of body weight.

    d. 1.2 gram of protein per kilogram of body weight.

45. The level associated with severe hypo-albuminemia is

    a. <2.5 g/dl.

    b. <3.5 g/dl.

    c. <4.0 g/dl.

    d. <6.0 g/dl.

46. An evaluation of nutritional status is indicated if, during a 6-month period, a patient has an unintentional loss of

    a. 5 lb.

    b. 10 lb.

    c. 3 lb.

    d. 7 lb.

47. Which of the following statements is correct concerning positioning?

    a. The use of donut-shaped devices relieves pressure on the sacrum.

    b. Turn the patient every 4 hours.

    c. Pullsheets, side rails, and overhead trapeze bars are effective devices to help reposition a patient.

    d. Keep the head of the bed elevated less than 60 degrees whenever possible.

48. Patients who are in sitting positions and able to shift their weight should be taught to change positions every

    a. 15 minutes.

    b. 30 minutes.

    c. 1 hour.

    d. 2 hours.

49. To decrease the risk of pressure ulcers when a patient is in a wheelchair, the thighs should be positioned

    a. elevated slightly above the hips.

    b. horizontal to the hips.

    c. slightly below the hips.

    d. with a pillow in-between.

50. To reduce pressure ulcer risk, an overlay mattress is used

    a. to replace a standard mattress for pressure reduction.

    b. to replace the complete hospital bed and frame for pressure relief.

    c. on top of the mattress to assist with pressure reduction.

    d. in conjunction with a specialty bed for pressure reduction.

51. A skin management measure that the clinician can do to improve the outcome of a patient at high risk for pressure ulcer development is

    a. use nonalkaline cleansing agents to preserve the acid mantle of the skin.

    b. ignore dry skin because it is part of the normal aging process and cannot be treated effectively.

    c. massage over bony prominences to increase circulation to the area.

    d. use disposable diapers that are plastic lined in managing patients with incontinence to keep linens clean.

CHAPTER 7

PRINCIPLES OF PRESSURE ULCER MANAGEMENT

CHAPTER OBJECTIVE

Upon completion of the chapter, the reader should be able to identify causes of pressure, anatomical locations for pressure ulcers, aspects of care that need to be included in the treatment plan, and alternative modalities used in pressure ulcer management.

LEARNING OBJECTIVES

After completion of the chapter, the reader will be able to

1. recognize causes of pressure and how they lead to injury.

2. list the three most common sites for pressure ulcers.

3. name two adjunctive therapies for pressure ulcer treatment.

INTRODUCTION

The incidence and prevalence of pressure ulcers varies from one clinical setting to another. The costs for treating and preventing these ulcers also varies by setting. Literature on the subject discusses the costs of treatment as well as their prevention. Data show that hospital-related costs are higher than skilled or home health costs due to nosocomial infections and other hospital-related complications. The cost of healing one pressure ulcer, including skilled long term care and hospital stay, was estimated at $2,731.00. The length of stay can be increased 3.5–5.0 times when a patient has a pressure ulcer. These are economic costs, but intangible costs associated with pressure ulcers make this problem more costly. When a clinician looks at these figures and then realizes that the majority of pressure ulcers are preventable, the cost figures become even more staggering. If a patient does develop a pressure ulcer, it is important to understand the available treatment options in order to provide quality, cost-effective care (Maklebust & Sieggreen, 2001).

In 2000, new objectives for the nation's health care system were developed at a national conference in Washington, DC. The inclusion of a pressure ulcer objective focuses the nation's attention and resources on this concern. The *Healthy People 2010* objective is to "reduce the proportion of nursing home residents with current diagnosis of pressure ulcers," the goal is to decrease prevalence by 50%, from 16% to 8% (http://health.gov/healthypeople).

PRESSURE ULCER FORMATION

Pressure ulcers are caused by soft tissue necrosis, which tends to develop when the soft tissue is compressed between a bony prominence and an external surface for a prolonged period. The two main determinants of pressure ulcer development are (1) intensity and duration of pressure and (2) tissue tolerance of the skin and its supporting structures. Pressure ulcers can be caused by a small amount of pressure over a long period of time or by a large amount of pressure over a short period of time. Extensive tissue damage can occur over the bone and other supporting tissues before the skin actually becomes broken, often appearing as an intact purple or red discolored area (see Figure 7-1). This discoloration of the area is referred to as the pressure gradient or "tip of the iceberg" effect. The damage to the fat and muscle tissues results because these tissues are less tolerant than skin to the decreased blood flow that transpires with pressure to the area. Additional factors lead to soft tissue destruction are shearing, friction, and excessive moisture (Maklebust & Sieggreen, 2001).

FIGURE 7-1
Mechanism of Pressure on Skin and Underlying Structures

Skin { Epidermis — Dermis —
Subcutaneous Fat
Deep Fascia —
Muscle —
Periosteum —
Bone —
Pressure

Reprinted with permission from *Pressure Ulcers: A Practical Nursing Reference for the Chronic Wound Care Environment*, 1995. Sugar Land, TX: Bertek Pharmaceuticals, Inc.

It is difficult to understand the true scope of the pressure ulcer problem, secondary to reporting difficulties and different ideas on what pressure ulcer formation means in terms of quality of care. A pressure ulcer problem does indeed exist, as evidenced by the rates of incidence and prevalence. Incidence is defined as the rate at which new cases of pressure ulcers develop; it is based on repeated observations of one specific population over a period of time. Prevalence refers to the number of pressure ulcer cases at any given point in time and involves only

one observation of one specific population. Prevalence rates can vary widely from patient population to settings to methodology. They are higher for elderly patients and patients who have spinal cord injuries or mobility problems. Rates also tend to be higher in long-term care facilities versus acute care settings, mostly because of the populations in these settings. The incidence rate in a facility is of great interest to all staff because it is an indicator of overall effectiveness of pressure ulcer prevention practices at a facility (Bryant, 2000).

Pressure ulcers occur most often over bony prominences. The sacrum, trochanters, ischial tuberosities (pressure points of the ischium), and calcaneus are the most frequent areas, but a pressure ulcer can develop anywhere pressure is exerted between two surfaces (see Figure 7-2). Table 7-1 identifies the most common sites for pressure ulcer formation as well as the frequency of ulceration per site (Bryant, 2000).

FIGURE 7-2
Pressure Ulcer

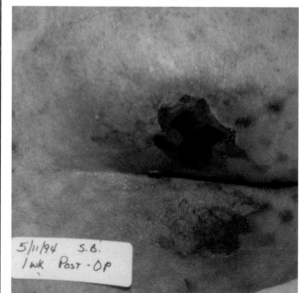

This is a 1-week postoperative photo of an 11-hour abdominal aortic aneurysm (AAA) repair. The patient was on a cooling blanket during surgery. Postoperatively, the patient refused any pressure-relieving device and only allowed limited turning.

TABLE 7-1
Common Sites for Pressure Ulcer Formation

SITE	FREQUENCY
Ischium	24%
Sacrum	23%
Trochanter	15%
Heel	8%
Lateral Malleolus	7%
Knee	6%
Iliac Crest	4%
Elbow	3%
Pretibial Crest	2%
Occiput	1%
Spinous Process	1%
Scapula	0.5%
Chin	0.5%

Adapted from Bryant, 2000.

Shearing

The force from shearing is another factor that leads to mechanical destruction of the skin and pressure ulcer formation. Shearing force is force that is parallel to the body. Shearing affects deep tissues and is caused by pulling the tissues attached to bone in one direction while the surface tissues remain stationary. Shearing reduces the time it takes for tissues to become ischemic and for tissue destruction, secondary to the occlusion of blood flow, to occur. A high enough shearing level can reduce by one-half the amount of pressure needed to produce vascular occlusion. Clinically, pressure ulcers that have a shearing component tend to have more of a triangular look to them than a rounded look and may have extensive tunneling or deep sinus tracts beneath them (Maklebust & Sieggreen, 2001).

Shearing effects are seen most often when patients require the head of the bed up and gravity pulls them down, which leads to the sliding motion that produces shearing. Shearing also takes place when patients either transfer themselves or are transferred by others and pulling or sliding of the

tissues occurs. Measures to decrease the ill effects of shearing were mentioned under "Mechanical Loading" and "Support Surfaces" in chapter 6, including

- If possible, keep the head of the bed elevated less than 30 degrees.

- Use pullsheets or other devices to lift the patient and avoid dragging the patient.

- Use overbed trapeze units, side rails, or other devices to allow the patient to assist with lifting.

- Use appropriate support surfaces to reduce shearing effects.

Careful evaluation of the patient's diagnosis can assist the clinician in recognizing potential problems with shearing so that measures may be instituted for prevention and treatment.

Friction

Friction is defined as surface damage caused by skin layers rubbing against another surface. Friction alone damages the epidermis and upper dermal layers but, in concert with gravity, can also lead to the detrimental effects of shearing. In the least severe case, friction abrades the epidermis and dermis similar to a mild burn. It is most evident in patients who are restless. Mild to moderate moisture, such as that caused by incontinence, exacerbates the effects of friction and leads to further skin breakdown (Bryant, 2000). Patients who are pulled along bed linens or who rub their extremities or heels repeatedly over bed linens are prone to mechanical destruction of cutaneous tissues from friction. The elderly population and patients who wear braces or other external devices that rub against the skin are at high risk for skin damage from friction. Measures to decrease friction (mentioned in chapter 6) include:

- lifting rather than pulling or dragging the patient

- using dry lubricants, such as cornstarch, or adherent dressings with slippery backings over at-risk skin to decrease the forces of friction (Maklebust & Sieggreen, 2001).

Moisture

The role of moisture in the formation of pressure ulcers has been well documented. Skin that has been excessively exposed to moisture eventually becomes waterlogged and macerated. The constant moisture breaks down connective tissue. Once the epidermis is macerated, it is easier for erosion to occur. With chronic exposure, degenerative changes take place and skin starts to slough off. Moist skin easily adheres to bed linens, and this adhesiveness worsens the risk of friction as the patient moves. Moist skin is five times more likely to break down with pressure ulcer formation than dry skin. Moisture is usually caused by urinary or fecal incontinence, perspiration, or wound drainage. A combination of fecal and urinary incontinence leads to chemical reactions that increase damage to the skin (Maklebust & Sieggreen, 2001). Specifically, the fecal enzymes become active in an alkaline environment. The pH rises when heat and occlusion are present, common findings in the perineal area, especially when adult briefs are used. Moist skin becomes more permeable and, therefore, more vulnerable to injury. The presence of fecal incontinence also increases the risk of secondary infection, especially to yeast (an opportunistic pathogen).

ASSESSMENT AND MEASUREMENT OF PRESSURE ULCERS

The risks associated with the development of pressure ulcers, as well as the tools utilized to measure these risks, were discussed in chapter 6. Pressure ulcer assessment and measurement is done in a similar fashion as for any other type of wound. A history must be obtained, and then the wound must be evaluated for anatomical location, stage, size, presence of tunneling or undermining, type of tissue in the wound bed, and drainage. The surrounding skin also needs to be assessed (see Figure 4-4 for an example of a wound assessment tool). The wound assessment and documentation principles outlined in chapter 4 also apply to pressure ulcer assessment.

Pressure ulcers may be evaluated with an array of wound assessment tools, but many lack some of the parameters necessary to give the clinician a picture of how the pressure ulcer looks or how it is responding to treatment.

Pressure Sore Status Tool

One tool that has been developed specifically for pressure ulcers is the Pressure Sore Status Tool or PSST (see Figure 7-3). This tool allows a quantitative evaluation of the pressure ulcer. There are 15 assessment items to evaluate, yet only 13 items are given scores. The assessment parameters location and shape are not given numerical scores but are checked off on the appropriate place on the PSST sheet. The items that are given a score include size, depth, edges, undermining, necrotic tissue type, necrotic tissue amount, exudate type and amount, skin color surrounding the wound, peripheral tissue edema and induration, granulation tissue, and epithelialization. Under each assessment item, there are five descriptors to choose from that clarify specific characteristics of the assessment item. After the 15 items have been evaluated, the scores are totaled to obtain a final assessment number, and this number is plotted along the pressure sore status continuum. Scores can range from 0–65 with 0 corresponding to tissue health, 13 to wound regeneration, and 65 to wound degeneration. Multiple scores can be plotted on the scale so that evaluation of overall wound progress can be made and appropriate measures taken in the treatment plan to promote healing.

Staging

With any evaluation of a pressure ulcer, the ulcer should be classified by the staging method that has been adopted by the *Agency for Health Care Research and Quality Pressure Ulcer Guideline Panels* (and accepted by Medicare). It is a four-stage system based on the tissue layers involved.

FIGURE 7-3 (*1 of 4*)
PRESSURE SORE STATUS TOOL
Instructions for Use

General Guidelines:

Fill out the attached rating sheet to assess a pressure sore's status after reading the definitions and methods of assessment described below. Evaluate once a week and whenever a change occurs in the wound. Rate according to each item by picking the response that best describes the wound and entering that score in the item score column for the appropriate date. When you have rated the pressure sore on all items, determine the total score by adding together the 13 item scores. The HIGHER the total score, the more severe the pressure sore status. Plot the total score on the Pressure Sore Status Continuum to determine progression of the wound.

Specific Instructions:

1. **Size:** Use a ruler to measure the longest and widest aspect of the wound surface in centimeters; multiply length x width.

2. **Depth:** Pick the depth, thickness, most appropriate to the wound using these descriptions:
    1 = tissues damaged but no break in skin surface.
    2 = superficial, abrasion, blister, or shallow crater. Even with and/or elevated above skin surface (e.g., hyperplasia).
    3 = deep crater with or without undermining of adjacent tissue.
    4 = visualization of tissue layers not possible due to necrosis.
    5 = supporting structures include tendon or joint capsule.

3. **Edges:**

Indistinct, diffuse	=	unable to clearly distinguish wound outline.
Attached	=	even or flush with wound base; **no** sides or walls present; flat.
Not attached	=	sides or walls **are** present; floor or base of wound is deeper than edge.
Rolled under, thickened	=	soft to firm and flexible to touch.
Hyperkeratosis	=	callous-like tissue formation around wound and at edges.
Fibrotic, scarred	=	hard, rigid to touch.

4. **Undermining:** Assess by inserting a cotton-tipped applicator under the wound edge; advance it as far as it will go without using undue force; raise the tip of the applicator so it may be seen or felt on the surface of the skin; mark the surface with a pen; measure the distance from the mark on the skin to the edge of the wound. Continue this process around the wound. Then use a transparent metric measuring guide with concentric circles divided into four (25%) pie-shaped quadrants to help determine percent of wound involved.

5. **Necrotic Tissue Type:** Pick the type of necrotic tissue that is **predominant** in the wound, according to color, consistency, and adherence, using this guide:

White/grey nonviable tissue	= may appear prior to wound opening; skin surface is white or grey.
Nonadherent, yellow slough	= thin, mucinous substance; scattered throughout wound bed; easily separated from wound tissue.
Loosely adherent, yellow slough	= thick, stringy, clumps of debris; attached to wound tissue.
Adherent, soft, black eschar	= soggy tissue; strongly attached to tissue in center or base of wound.
Firmly adherent, hard, black eschar	= firm, crusty tissue; strongly attached to wound base **and** edges (like a hard scab).

6. **Necrotic Tissue Amount:** Use a transparent metric measuring guide with concentric circles divided into four (25%) pie-shaped quadrants to help determine percent of wound involved.

7. **Exudate Type:** Some dressings interact with wound drainage to produce a gel or trap liquid. Before assessing exudate type, gently cleanse the wound with normal saline solution or water. Pick the exudate type that is **predominant** in the wound according to color and consistency, using this guide:

Bloody	= thin, bright red.
Serosanguineous	= thin, watery pale red to pink.
Serous	= thin, watery, clear.
Purulent	= thin or thick, opaque tan to yellow.
Foul purulent	= thick, opaque yellow to green with offensive odor.

FIGURE 7-3 *(2 of 4)*

8. **Exudate Amount:** Use a transparent metric measuring guide with concentric circles divided into four (25%) pie-shaped quadrants to help determine percent of dressing involved with exudate. Use this guide:

    None   = wound tissues dry.

    Scant   = wound tissues moist; no measurable exudate.

    Small   = wound tissues wet; moisture evenly distributed in wound; drainage involves ≤25% dressing.

    Moderate = wound tissues saturated; drainage may or may not be evenly distributed in wound; drainage involves >25% but ≤75% dressing.

    Large   = wound tissues bathed in fluid; drainage freely expressed; may or may not be evenly distributed in wound; drainage involves >75% of dressing.

9. **Skin Color Surrounding Wound:** Assess tissues within 4 cm of wound edge. Dark-skinned persons show the colors "bright red" and "dark red" as a deepening of normal ethnic skin color or a purple hue. As healing occurs in dark-skinned persons, the new skin is pink and may never darken.

10. **Peripheral Tissue Edema:** Assess tissues within 4 cm of wound edge. Nonpitting edema appears as skin that is shiny and taut. Identify pitting edema by firmly pressing a finger down into the tissues and waiting for 5 seconds; on release of pressure, tissues fail to resume previous position and an indentation appears. Crepitus is accumulation of air or gas in tissues. Use a transparent metric measuring guide to determine how far edema extends beyond the wound.

11. **Peripheral Tissue Induration:** Assess tissues within 4 cm of wound edge. Induration is abnormal firmness of tissues with margins. Assess by gently pinching the tissues. Induration results in an inability to pinch the tissues. Use a transparent metric measuring guide with concentric circles divided into four (25%) pie-shaped quadrants to determine percent of wound and area involved.

12. **Granulation Tissue:** Granulation tissue is the growth of small blood vessels and connective tissue to fill in full thickness wounds. Tissue is healthy when bright, beefy red, shiny and granular with a velvety appearance. Poor vascular supply appears as pale pink or blanched to dull, dusky red color.

13. **Epithelialization:** Epithelialization is the process of epidermal resurfacing and appears as pink or red skin. In partial thickness wounds it can occur throughout the wound bed as well as from the wound edges. In full-thickness wounds it occurs from the edges only. Use a transparent metric measuring guide with concentric circles divided into four (25%) pie-shaped quadrants to help determine percent of wound involved and to measure the distance the epithelial tissue extends into the wound.

FIGURE 7-3 *(3 of 4)*
PRESSURE SORE STATUS TOOL

NAME _____

Complete the rating sheet to assess pressure sore status. Evaluate each item by picking the response that best describes the wound and entering the score in the item score column for the appropriate date.

Location: Anatomic site. Circle, identify right (R) or left (L) and use "X" to mark site on body diagrams.

____ Sacrum & coccyx	____ Lateral ankle
____ Trochanter	____ Medial ankle
____ Ischial tuberosity	____ Heel ____ Other site

Shape: Overall wound pattern; assess by observing perimeter and depth. Circle and **date** appropriate description.

____ Irregular	____ Linear or elongated
____ Round/oval	____ Bowl/boat
____ Square/rectangle	____ Butterfly ____ Other shape

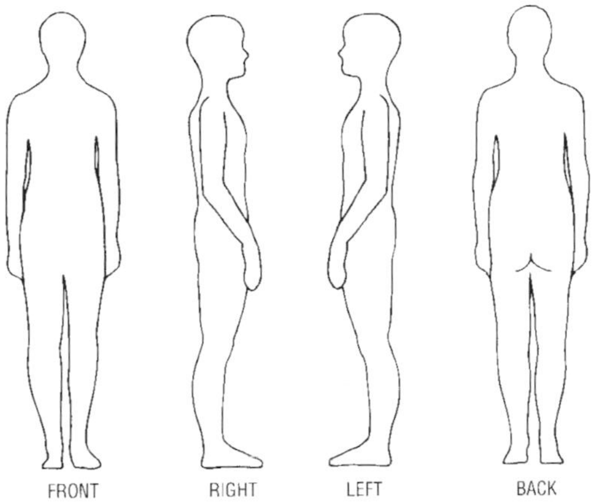

FRONT   RIGHT   LEFT   BACK

ITEM	ASSESSMENT	DATE SCORE	DATE SCORE	DATE SCORE
1. Size	1 = Length x width <4 sq cm 2 = Length x width 4 – 16 sq cm 3 = Length x width 16.1 – 36 sq cm 4 = Length x width 36.1 – 80 sq cm 5 = Length x width >80 sq cm			
2. Depth	1 = Nonblanchable erythema on intact skin 2 = Partial thickness skin loss involving epidermis and/or dermis 3 = Full thickness skin loss involving damage or necrosis of subcutaneous tissue; may extend down to but not through underlying fascia; and/or mixed partial and full thickness and/or tissue layers obscured by granulation tissue 4 = Obscured by necrosis 5 = Full thickness skin loss with extensive destruction, tissue necrosis or damage to muscle, bone or supporting structures			
3. Edges	1 = Indistinct, diffuse, none clearly visible 2 = Distinct, outline clearly visible, attached, even with wound base 3 = Well-defined, not attached to wound base 4 = Well-defined, not attached to base, rolled under, thickened 5 = Well-defined, fibrotic, scarred or hyperkeratotic			
4. Undermining	1 = Undermining <2 cm in any area 2 = Undermining 2 – 4 cm involving <50% wound margins 3 = Undermining 2 – 4 cm involving >50% wound margins 4 = Undermining >4 cm in any area 5 = Tunneling and/or sinus tract formation			
5. Necrotic Tissue Type	1 = None visible 2 = White/grey nonviable tissue and/or nonadherent yellow slough 3 = Loosely adherent yellow slough 4 = Adherent, soft, black eschar 5 = Firmly adherent, hard, black eschar			
6. Necrotic Tissue Amount	1 = None visible 2 = <25% of wound bed covered 3 = 25% to 50% of wound covered 4 = >50% and <75% of wound covered 5 = 75% to 100% of wound covered			

FIGURE 7-3 *(4 of 4)*
PRESSURE SORE STATUS TOOL

ITEM	ASSESSMENT	DATE SCORE	DATE SCORE	DATE SCORE
7. Exudate Type	1 = None or bloody 2 = Serosanguineous: thin, watery, pale red/pink 3 = Serous: thin, watery, clear 4 = Purulent: thin or thick, opaque, tan/yellow 5 = Foul purulent: thick, opaque, yellow/green with odor			
8. Exudate Amount	1 = None 2 = Scant 3 = Small 4 = Moderate 5 = Large			
9. Skin Color Surrounding Wound	1 = Pink or normal for ethnic group 2 = Bright red and/or blanches to touch 3 = White or grey pallor or hypopigmented 4 = Dark red or purple and/or nonblanchable 5 = Black or hyperpigmented			
10. Peripheral Tissue Edema	1 = Minimal swelling around wound 2 = Nonpitting edema extends < 4 cm around wound 3 = Nonpitting edema extends ≥ 4 cm around wound 4 = Pitting edema extends < 4 cm around wound 5 = Crepitus and/or pitting edema extends ≥ 4 cm			
11. Peripheral Tissue Induration	1 = Minimal firmness around wound 2 = Induration < 2 cm around wound 3 = Induration 2 – 4 cm extending < 50% around wound 4 = Induration 2 – 4 cm extending ≥ 50% around wound 5 = Induration > 4 cm in any area			
12. Granulation Tissue	1 = Skin intact or partial thickness wound 2 = Bright, beefy red; 75% to 100% of wound filled and/or tissue overgrowth 3 = Bright, beefy red; < 75% and > 25% of wound filled 4 = Pink, and/or dull, dusky red and/or fills ≤ 25% of wound 5 = No granulation tissue present			
13. Epithelialization	1 = 100% wound covered, surface intact 2 = 75% to < 100% wound covered and/or epithelial tissue extends > 0.5 cm into wound bed 3 = 50% to < 75% wound covered and/or epithelial tissue extends to < 0.5 cm into wound bed 4 = 25% to < 50% wound covered 5 = < 25% wound covered			
TOTAL SCORE				
SIGNATURE				

PRESSUE SORE STATUS CONTINUUM

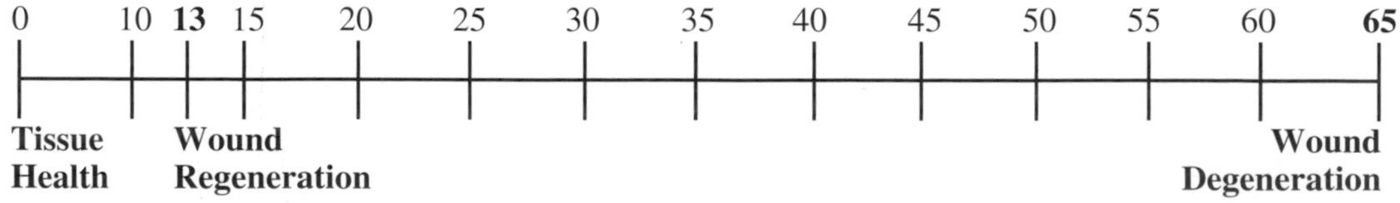

```
0      10  13  15     20      25      30      35      40      45      50      55      60      65
|------|---|--|-------|-------|-------|-------|-------|-------|-------|-------|-------|-------|
Tissue     Wound                                                            Wound
Health     Regeneration                                                     Degeneration
```

Plot the total score on the Pressure Score Status Continuum by putting an "X" on the line and the date beneath the line. Plot multiple scores with their dates to see at-a-glance regeneration or degeneration of the wound.

The system was derived from previous staging systems proposed by Shea (1975), the Wound, Ostomy, and Continence Nurses Society (WOCN, 1988) and the National Pressure Ulcer Advisory Panel (NPUAP, 1989 Consensus Conference and a 1998 revision of Stage I definition). This staging method looks at the layers of tissue involved from the opening of the wound down to the depth. When the depth of the wound cannot be visualized secondary to a necrotic base, the wound cannot be staged (see Figures 7-4 & 7-5). Once the necrotic base is cleared and the wound base is visualized, the wound can be staged. The only exception is in long-term care, for which Minimum Data Sheet (MDS) forms have not been adjusted to accommodate for the inability to stage a wound with eschar. These wounds with eschar are classified as Stage IV until the base can be visualized. The following definitions describe the four stages.

Stage I: An observable pressure-related alteration of intact skin whose indicators, as compared to the adjacent or opposite area on the body, may include changes in one or more of the following conditions: skin temperature (warmth or coolness), tissue consistency (firm or boggy feel),

FIGURE 7-5
Unstageable Pressure Ulcer #2

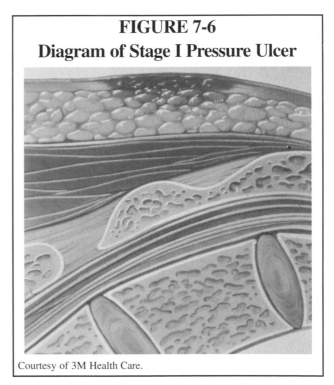

Pressure ulcer that is not able to be staged
Courtesy of 3M Health Care.

and sensation (pain, itching). The ulcer appears as a defined area of persistent redness in lightly pigmented skin; in darker skin tones, the ulcer may appear with persistent red, blue, or purple hues (see Figures 7-6 & 7-7).

FIGURE 7-6
Diagram of Stage I Pressure Ulcer

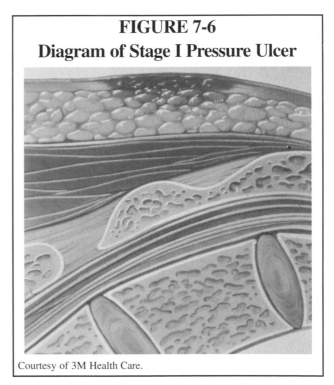

Courtesy of 3M Health Care.

FIGURE 7-4
Unstageable Pressure Ulcer #1

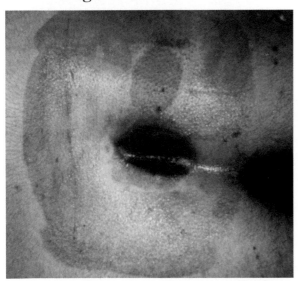

Pressure ulcer that is not able to be staged
Courtesy of 3M Health Care.

FIGURE 7-7
Stage I Pressure Ulcer

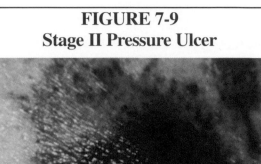

Courtesy of 3M Health Care.

Stage II: Partial-thickness skin loss involving the epidermis and/or dermis. The ulcer is superficial and presents clinically as an abrasion, blister, or shallow crater (see Figures 7-8 & 7-9).

FIGURE 7-8
Diagram of Stage II Pressure Ulcer

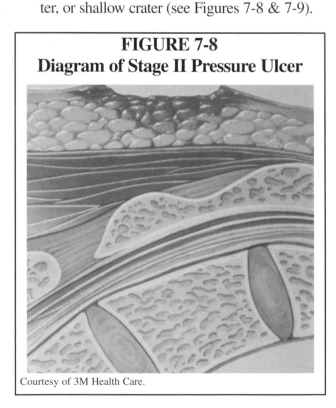

Courtesy of 3M Health Care.

FIGURE 7-9
Stage II Pressure Ulcer

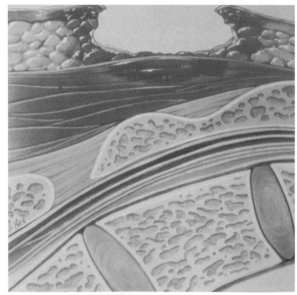

Courtesy of 3M Health Care.

Stage III: Full-thickness skin loss involving damage or necrosis of subcutaneous tissue that may extend down to, but not through, the underlying fascia. The ulcer presents clinically as a deep crater with or without undermining of adjacent tissue (see Figures 7-10 & 7-11).

FIGURE 7-10
Diagram of Stage III Pressure Ulcer

Courtesy of 3M Health Care.

FIGURE 7-11
Stage III Pressure Ulcer

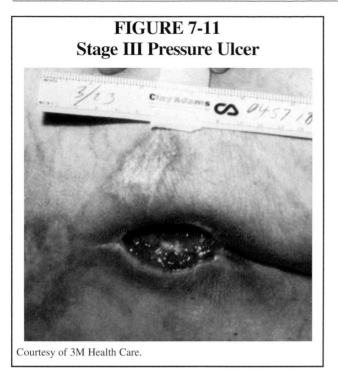

Courtesy of 3M Health Care.

Stage IV: Full-thickness skin loss with extensive destruction, tissue necrosis, or damage to muscle, bone, or supporting structures — for example, a tendon or joint capsule (see Figures 7-12, 7-13, & 7-14).

FIGURE 7-12
Diagram of Stage IV Pressure Ulcer

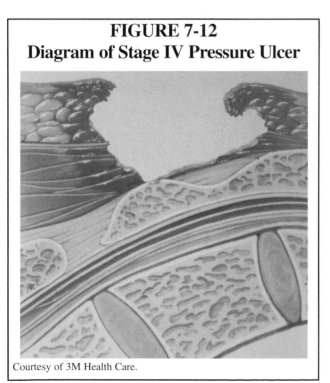

Courtesy of 3M Health Care.

FIGURE 7-13
Stage IV Pressure Ulcer

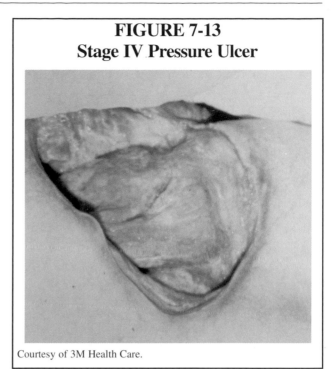

Courtesy of 3M Health Care.

FIGURE 7-14
Stage IV Pressure Ulcer with Necrotic Tissue

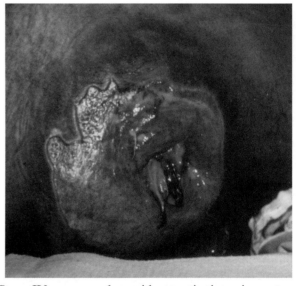

Stage IV pressure ulcer with necrotic tissue in center.

There is another classification of pressure ulcer called a *closed pressure ulcer*. In this situation, the lesion is closed (as the name implies) but is caused by the same pathological process. This classification of pressure ulcer many times looks harmless; however, underneath the surface, a potentially lethal lesion is forming whereby ischemic necrosis in subcutaneous fat occurs without skin ulceration. The resulting cavity is filled with necrotic debris. As the inflammatory process continues, the skin eventually ruptures, resulting in a superficial-looking defect with an extensive amount of drainage and damage below. These types of ulcers often involve the pelvic region of healthy spinal cord–injured patients who are confined to wheelchairs. These ulcers are not staged, because it is impossible to know the extent of damage until the wound is opened by surgical incision. Treatment for closed pressure ulcers includes surgical intervention and closure with a muscle rotation flap (Maklebust & Sieggreen, 2001).

PRESSURE ULCER TREATMENT AND PREVENTION

Pressure ulcers have many of the same treatment considerations as other wounds but, as their name implies, pressure must be addressed. The risk factors for pressure ulcer development need to be continually monitored, and pressure ulcer prevention principles need to be instituted. Devices, support surfaces, and patient positioning needs to be utilized for pressure reduction and relief. If a device is able to redistribute the pressure over a bony prominence to a larger surface, then the chance for pressure ulcer formation over that bony prominence is decreased. Needed support surfaces should be evaluated not only for the patient's bed but for the patient's chair and seating environments as well. Without pressure reduction or relief practices, the wound will not respond to therapy no matter what type of topical treatment is instituted. Following the recommendations and algorithms designated in the *AHCPR Clinical Practice Guidelines: Treatment of Pressure Ulcers* can guide the clinician in the standard of care for pressure ulcer management.

Nutrition

Studies have linked malnutrition to the formation of pressure ulcers; therefore, nutritional status has been targeted as one of the fundamental aspects to consider with regard to pressure ulcer treatment and prevention. Nutritional assessment and management have the goal of ensuring that the diet of a patient with a pressure ulcer contains nutrients adequate to support healing. The nutritional algorithm from the *AHCPR Clinical Practice Guidelines: Treatment of Pressure Ulcers* can assist in meeting this goal (see Figure 7-15).

Here are the main points to consider regarding nutrition

- Ensure adequate dietary intake to prevent malnutrition to the extent that is compatible with the patient's wishes.

- Perform an abbreviated nutritional assessment, as defined by the Nutrition Screening Initiative, at least once every 3 months for individuals at risk for malnutrition (see Figure 7-16). These include individuals who are unable to take food by mouth or who experience an involuntary change in weight. (The Nutritional Screening Initiative is a publication offering guidelines to health care providers who assist in the nutritional management of the older population.)

- Encourage dietary intake or supplementation for the malnourished patient with a pressure ulcer. If dietary intake continues to be inadequate, impractical, or impossible, nutritional support should be used to place the patient into positive nitrogen balance. (Approximately 30–35 calories/kg/day and 1.25–1.50 grams of protein/kg/day.).

- Provide vitamin and mineral supplements if deficiencies are confirmed or suspected (see Figure 7-17) (AHCPR, 1994).

It is always an excellent idea to consult a dietitian for assistance with recommendations on nutritional evaluation tools and suggestions for dietary supplementation for at-risk or malnourished patients.

FIGURE 7-15
Nutritional Assessment and Support

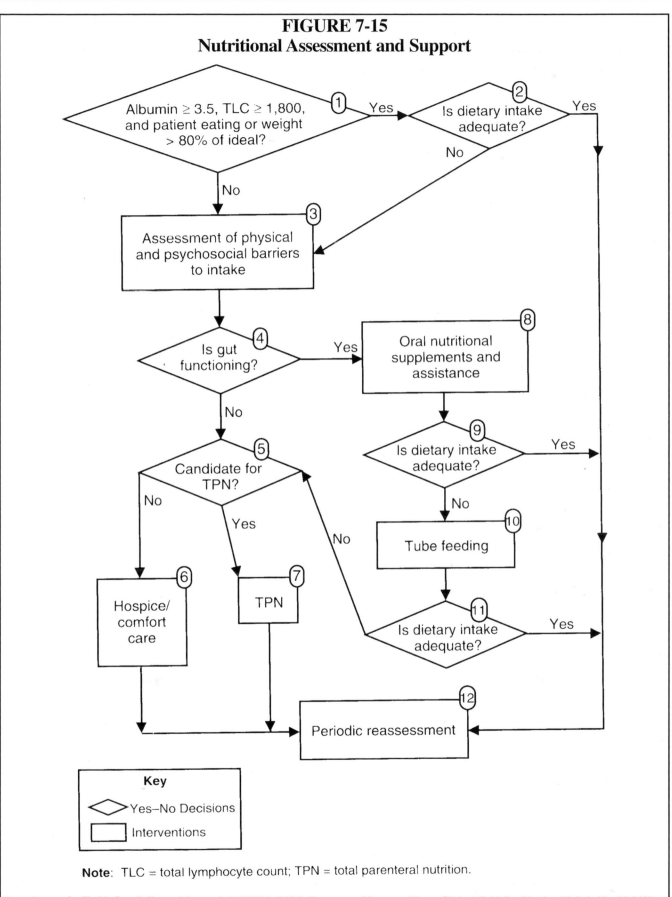

Note: TLC = total lymphocyte count; TPN = total parenteral nutrition.

FIGURE 7-16
Sample Nutritional Assessment Guide for Patients with Pressure Ulcers

Patient Name: _____   Date: _____ Time: _____

To be filled out for all patients at risk on initial evaluation and every 12 weeks thereafter, as indicated. Trends will document the efficacy of nutritional support therapy.

Protein Compartments

Somatic:

Current Weight (kg)	_____
Previous Weight (kg)	_____ (_____date)
Percent Change in Weight	_____
Height (cm)	_____
Height/Weight	_____
Current Body Mass Index (BMI)	_____ [wt/(ht)^2]
Previous BMI	_____ (_____date)
Percent Change in BMI	_____

Visceral:

Serum Albumin   _____
    (Normal $\geq$ 3.5 mg/dL)
Total Lymphocyte Count (TLC)   _____ (optional)
    (White Blood Cell count x percent Lymphocytes/100)

Guide to TLC:
- Immune competence $\geq$ 1,800 mm^3
- Immunity partly impaired   < 1,800 but $\geq$ 900 mm^3
- Anergy   < 900 mm^3

State of Hydration

24-Hour Intake _____ mL   24-Hour Output _____mL

Note: Thirst, tongue dryness in non-mouth-breathers and tenting of cervical skin may indicate dehydration. Jugular vein distension may indicate overhydration.

Estimated Nutritional Requirement

Estimated Nonprotein Calories (NPC)_____/kg   Estimated Protein _____ (g/kg)

Actual NPC   _____ /kg   Actual Protein _____ (g/kg)

Recommendations/Plan

1.

2.

3.

4.

FIGURE 7-17
Oral and Cutaneous Signs of Vitamin or Mineral Deficiencies

Clinical Signs (by Site)	Deficiency(ies)
Oral Cavity	
Cheilosis and angular stomatitis	Vitamin B_2
Glossitis (i.e., pink or magenta discoloration with loss of villi)	Multiple B vitamins
Eyes	
Scleral changes	Vitamin A
Bitot's spots	Vitamin A
Face	
Seborrhea-like dryness and redness of nasolabial fold and eyebrows	Zinc
Upper Extremities	
Purplish blotches on lightly traumatized areas (due to capillary fragility and subepithelial hemorrhages)	Vitamin C
Extreme transparency of skin of hands ("cellophane skin")	Vitamin C
Abdomen/Buttocks	
Waxy, perifollicular hyperkeratosis	Vitamin A
Lower Extremities	
Superficial flaking of epidermis, large flakes of dandruff	Essential fatty acids
Cracks in skin between islands of hyperkeratosis:	
■ Pigmented	Nicotinamide (niacinamide)
■ Nonpigmented	Vitamin A

Note: These manifestations may be seen in disease processes other than vitamin deficiencies. If the cause is in fact a deficiency, clinical improvement should be evident 4 weeks after supplementation is begun.

From Agency for Health Care Policy and Research (AHCPR). (1994). *Treatment of Pressure Ulcers.* Clinical Guideline Number 15, Pub. No. 95-0652. National Library of Medicine. Retrieved April 6, 2004 from http://hstat.nlm.nih.gov/

Managing Tissue Loads and Support Surfaces

The pressure ulcer prevention information in chapter 6 opened the discussion on the use of support surfaces and their benefits to a patient who is at risk for development of pressure ulcers. Support surfaces are also utilized for the treatment of pressure ulcers. The selection of a support surface should be based on the therapeutic benefit associated with the surface. The support surface choice should take into consideration the clinical condition of the patient, the characteristics of the care setting, and the characteristics of the support surface (see Figure 7-18). Additional aspects to consider when choosing the correct support surface include ease of use, requirements for maintenance, cost, and patient preference.

FIGURE 7-18
Selected Characteristics for Classes of Support Surfaces

Performance Characteristics	Support Devices					
	Air-Fluidized	Low-Air-Loss	Alternating Air	Static Flotation (air or water)	Foam	Standard Mattress
Increased support area	Yes	Yes	Yes	Yes	Yes	No
Low moisture retention	Yes	Yes	No	No	No	No
Reduced heat accumulation	Yes	Yes	No	No	No	No
Shear reduction	Yes	?	Yes	Yes	No	No
Pressure reduction	Yes	Yes	Yes	Yes	Yes	No
Dynamic	Yes	Yes	Yes	No	No	No
Cost per day	High	High	Moderate	Low	Low	Low

From *Treatment of Pressure Ulcers.* U.S. Department of Health and Human Services, 1994.

Additional points to consider regarding the use of support surfaces include

- Assess all patients with existing pressure ulcers to determine their risk of developing additional pressure ulcers. If a patient remains at risk, use a pressure-reducing surface.

- Use a static support surface when a patient can assume a variety of positions without bearing weight on a pressure ulcer and without bottoming out.

- Use a dynamic support surface when the patient cannot assume a variety of positions without bearing weight on a pressure ulcer, when the patient fully compresses the static support surface, or when the pressure ulcer does not show evidence of healing.

- In a patient with large Stage III or Stage IV pressure ulcers on multiple turning surfaces, a low-air-loss bed or an air-fluidized bed may be indicated.

- When excess moisture on intact skin is a potential source of maceration and skin breakdown, use a support surface that provides airflow, which can be important for drying the skin and preventing additional pressure ulcers.

For patients who are in the sitting position for periods of time with limited mobility, the following points should be noted

- Ensure that a patient who has a pressure ulcer on a sitting surface avoids sitting. If pressure on the ulcer can be relieved, limited sitting may be allowed.

- Consider postural alignment, distribution of weight, balance, stability, and pressure relief when positioning sitting patients.

- Reposition the sitting patient at least once every hour so that the points under pressure are shifted . If this schedule cannot be kept or is inconsistent with overall treatment goals, return the patient to bed. Patients who are able, should be taught to shift their weight every 15 minutes.

- Select a cushion based on the specific needs of the patient who requires pressure reduction in a sitting position. Avoid donut-type devices.

- Develop a written plan for the use of positioning devices (AHCPR, 1994).

PRESSURE ULCER CARE

The treatment of pressure ulcers should always follow a few simple principles

- Debride necrotic tissue, as needed, on initial and subsequent visits.

- Cleanse the wound initially and with each dressing change.

- Prevent, diagnose, and treat infection.

- Use a dressing that keeps the ulcer bed continuously moist and the surrounding tissue dry.

- Assess ulcer healing and the efficacy of the basic treatment plan at least weekly.

- Adjust the basic treatment plan if the ulcer is not healing.

- Refer the patient for adjunctive therapies if the wound is slow to respond to treatment or shows no healing progress. Refer to chapter 12 for more information on adjunctive therapies.

Specific Pressure Ulcer Treatments

The use of debridement, wound cleansing, types of available dressings, and management of infection are covered in more detail in chapter 9. The principles of these treatments are covered here.

Debridement

- Remove devitalized tissue in pressure ulcers when appropriate for the patient's condition and consistent with patient goals.

- Select a method of debridement most appropriate to the patient's condition and goals. Mechanical, enzymatic, or autolytic debridement techniques may be used when drainage or the area or removal of devitalized tissue is not clinically urgent. If there is an urgent need for debridement, such as with advancing cellulitis or sepsis, sharp debridement should be used.

- Use clean, dry dressings for 8–24 hours after sharp debridement associated with bleeding; then reinstitute moist dressings. Clean, dry dressings may be used in conjunction with mechanical or enzymatic debridement techniques.

- Heel ulcers with dry eschar need not be debrided if they do not have edema, erythema, fluctuance, or drainage. Assess these wounds daily to monitor for pressure ulcer complications that would require debridement.

- Prevent or manage pain associated with debridement.

Wound Cleansing

- Cleanse wounds initially and at each dressing change.

- Use minimal mechanical force when cleansing the ulcer with gauze, cloth, or sponges.

- Do not clean ulcer wounds with skin cleansers or antiseptic agents, such as povodine iodine, iodophor, sodium hypochlorite solution (Dakin's solution), hydrogen peroxide, or acetic acid.

- Use normal saline solution for cleansing most pressure ulcers.

- Use enough irrigation pressure to enhance wound cleansing without causing trauma to the wound bed. Safe and effective ulcer irrigation pressures range from 4–15 psi.

- Consider whirlpool treatment for cleansing pressure ulcers that contain thick exudate, slough, or necrotic tissue. Discontinue whirlpool when the ulcer is clean.

Dressings

- Use a dressing that keeps the ulcer bed continuously moist. Wet-to-dry dressings should be used only for debridement and are not considered continuously moist saline dressings.

- Use clinical judgment to select a type of moist wound dressing suitable for the ulcer. Keep in mind the amount of drainage from the wound, the characteristics of the wound bed, the patient setting, cost, frequency desired, who will change the dressing, and availability of the dressing.

- Choose a dressing that keeps the surrounding intact skin dry while keeping the ulcer bed moist.

- Choose a dressing that controls exudate but does not desiccate the ulcer bed.

- Consider caregiver time when selecting a dressing.

- Eliminate wound dead space by loosely filling all cavities with dressing material. Avoid over-packing the wound.

Infection Control

- When treating pressure ulcers, follow body substance isolation precautions or an equivalent system appropriate for the health care setting and the patient's condition.

- Use clean gloves for each patient. When treating multiple ulcers on the same patient, attend to the most contaminated ulcer last. Remove gloves and wash hands between patients.

- Use sterile instruments to debride pressure ulcers.

- As long as dressing procedures comply with institutional infection control guidelines, use clean dressings, rather than sterile ones, to treat pressure ulcers.

- Use clean dressings in the home setting. Disposal of contaminated dressings in the home should be done in a manner consistent with local regulations.

(AHCPR, 1994)

ADJUNCTIVE THERAPIES

Several new wound care modalities have been introduced for the treatment of pressure ulcers, including electrical stimulation, growth factors, hyperbaric oxygen, cultured epithelium, and ultrasound therapy. Adjunctive therapies continue to expand as technology advances and the understanding of wound healing and infection improves. Although existing research supporting these therapies is limited, new research continues. The controversial nature of these therapies also sparks new ideas and opens new doors. The focus is supporting the patient and promoting wound healing in various ways. The challenge is that no two wounds are alike and each presents a problem unique to the individual patient. Brief descriptions of the modalities appear below. Note that the only treatment that is recommended by the *AHCPR Clinical Practice Guidelines* is electrical stimulation.

Electrical Stimulation: use of electrical waveforms in wound healing to increase blood flow, stimulate collagen formation and phagocytosis, and enhance growth of fibroblasts and keratinocytes. The process is noninvasive and can be performed through clothing and dressings. Three types of electrical waveforms are used: low-intensity direct current, high-voltage pulsed current, and pulsed electrical stimulation.

Growth Factors: use of the body's own growth factors to promote new granulation tissue and new skin to cover the wound. A variety of growth factors exist, such as platelet-derived growth factor, fibroblast growth factor, transforming growth factor alpha, transforming growth factor beta, interleukins, and epidermal growth factors. The growth factor most frequently utilized is platelet-derived growth factor, whereby a patient's blood is drawn and sent to a laboratory where the platelet growth factors are isolated and placed into a solution for the patient or clinician to administer topically to the wound.

Hyperbaric Oxygen: utilization of 100% oxygen under a pressure that is greater than one atmosphere. The patient is placed into a chamber that can deliver hyperbaric oxygen. As the patient breathes this oxygen, the atmospheric pressure is increased so that the oxygen is dissolved into the patient's plasma at a higher concentration than it would be dissolved at sea level. The supersaturation of hemoglobin leads to a greater supply of oxygen to the tissues. This increased oxygen is thought to improve healing rate.

Cultured Epithelium: use of cultured cells in vitro to produce viable epithelial sheets that can be used in the treatment of skin ulcers. This technique may be more useful in the management of burn injuries where split-thickness skin grafting is utilized. Minimal data is available on the use of this modality with pressure ulcers.

Ultrasound: use of high frequency sound waves generated by the oscillation of a crystal in a transducer. Ultrasound therapy can be given in either a continuous mode or a pulsed interrupted mode. The passage of the waveform across the cell wall is thought to lead to a change in the diffusion rate and the permeability of the cell membrane and to influence the wound healing trajectory.

(Maklebust & Sieggreen, 2001)

OPERATIVE REPAIR OF PRESSURE ULCERS

Operative repair of pressure ulcers is usually reserved for Stage III and Stage IV ulcers that have not responded to more conservative treatment options. Surgical repair enables rapid skin closure and repair. Before surgical intervention is instituted, several criteria need to be addressed. These criteria include the patient's medical condition and nutritional status, the likelihood that the operation will enhance the patient's functional status, and the patient's ability to tolerate the surgical procedure and the postoperative recovery process. Discussion also needs to include the patient's concerns regarding treatment goals, risk of recurrence, rehabilitation outcomes, personal preferences, and quality of life issues.

Typical operative procedures include direct closure, skin grafting, skin flaps, musculocutaneous flaps, and free flaps. Definitions of various types of operative procedures are listed here.

Delay of Flaps: development and transfer of a flap to a recipient site in more than one step to ensure its vascular supply.

Direct Closure: direct primary closure with sutures, which stretches the skin and creates tension that frequently leads to dehiscence and therefore is seldom used except for small, superficial ulcers.

Free Flap: procedure involving a muscle-type flap in which the vein and artery are disconnected at the donor site and reconnected to the vessels at the recipient site with the aid of a microscope.

Muscle Flap: procedure in which a known muscle and its vascular supply (either intact or reestablished) are moved into a defect.

Musculocutaneous: procedure in which a muscle combined with a portion flap of overlying skin having an intact vascular supply is moved. The portion of skin overlying the muscle is fed by perforators within the muscle.

Sensate Flap: procedure in which muscle, skin, and a sensory nerve are moved. The sensory nerve provides feeling to the flap.

Skin Flap: procedure in which a section of skin and associated subcutaneous tissue from one part of the body are moved to another, with the vascular supply maintained for nourishment. The vascular attachment can be the original vessel, rotated along with the flap; changed from one part of the flap to another; or reestablished by microvascular anastomoses once it has been placed in the new location.

Skin Graft: procedure in which a segment of dermis and a portion of epidermis are moved. The graft is completely separated from its blood supply and donor site and moved to a recipient site. Skin grafts contain varying portions of epidermis and dermis and can be full thickness or partial thickness, depending on how much dermis is included in the graft.

Tissue Expansion: surgical technique during which an expandable device is placed beneath viable skin. The device is expanded with serial injections of saline solution and, when the skin has stretched, it is moved to cover a nearby defect.

V-Y Advancement: procedure that derives its name from the appearance of the postoperative wound. After an incision is made in the shape of a "V," the apex of the "V" is closed by advancing the central portion. This leaves a scar that looks like a "Y."

Surgical repair may require only one of or a combination of these procedures. Selection of the type of repair depends on the location of the ulcer, history of prior ulcerations and surgery, the patient's mobility status, daily routines, and other medical conditions.

Operative procedures vary in length from 1–3 hours and can result in blood loss of up to 1,500 ml. Patients who have medical conditions that could worsen with the stress of surgery and the potential blood loss are not good surgical candidates (AHCPR, 1994).

Postoperative care of the patient involves maintaining circulation to the grafts and prevention of infection. Patients are usually kept immobile for 2 weeks and are usually placed on a low-air-loss or air-fluidized support surface for pressure relief. Turning the patient should be done with caution to avoid tension on the suture line and to avoid the effects of friction and shearing on the surgical site. Patients should be lifted, rather than slid, across the surface of the bed. The surgical site should be inspected for any skin changes, such as pallor or cyanosis, that could indicate a problem with circulation. Incision sites are carefully cleaned with nor-

mal saline solution to keep them free from contamination and drainage.

Approximately 2 weeks after surgery, the patient can begin increased activity with some sitting time allowed. Protocols of the health care facility or physician should be followed. The surgical site should be inspected each time the patient has had any pressure to the area. An emphasis on patient education is a must with surgical intervention because the recurrence rates vary depending on patient compliance with skin care and pressure-relief practices (Maklebust & Sieggreen, 2001).

EDUCATION

Health care facilities and agencies are responsible for formulating and implementing educational programs that are designed to improve the clinician's knowledge base concerning the treatment of pressure ulcers. The clinician can then convert that knowledge into effective pressure ulcer treatment programs. The outcomes for these programs should have an emphasis on preventing new pressure ulcers, promoting healing, and preventing deterioration in existing pressure ulcers. The *AHCPR Clinical Practice Guidelines: Treatment of Pressure Ulcers* lists several recommendations that should be included in developing and implementing an educational program on pressure ulcers. Here are some of those recommendations

- Design, develop, and implement educational programs for patients, caregivers, and health care providers that reflect a continuum of care. The program should begin with a structured, comprehensive, and organized approach to prevention and should culminate in effective treatment protocols that promote healing as well as prevent recurrence. Emphasize the need for accurate, consistent, and uniform assessment, description, and documentation of the extent of tissue damage.

- Develop educational programs that target appropriate health care providers, patients, family members, and caregivers. Identify those responsible for pressure ulcer treatment and describe each person's role. The degree of participation expected should be appropriate to the audience. Present information at an appropriate level for the target audience to maximize retention and ensure carryover into practice. Use principles of adult learning (for example, explanation, demonstration, questioning, group discussion, and drills).

- Involve the patient and caregiver, when possible, in pressure ulcer treatment and prevention strategies and options. Include information on pain, discomfort, possible outcomes, and duration of treatment, if known. Encourage the patient to actively participate in, and comply with, decisions regarding pressure ulcer prevention and treatment.

- Include the following information when developing an educational program on the treatment of pressure ulcers
  — etiology and pathology
  — risk factors
  — uniform terminology for stages of tissue damage based on specific classification
  — principles of wound healing
  — principles of nutritional support with regard to tissue integrity
  — individualized program of skin care
  — principles of cleansing and infection control
  — principles of postoperative care, including positioning and support surfaces
  — principles of prevention to reduce recurrence
  — product selection (such as categories and uses of support surfaces, dressings, topical antibiotics, or other agents)
  — effects or influence of the physical and mechanical environment on the pressure ulcer and strategies for management
  — mechanisms for accurate documentation and monitoring of pertinent data, including treatment interventions and healing progress.

- Update educational programs on an ongoing and regular basis to integrate new knowledge, techniques, or technologies.

- Evaluate the effectiveness of an educational program in terms of measurable outcomes: implementing of guideline recommendations, healing of existing ulcers, reducing the incidence of new or recurrent ulcers, and preventing the deterioration of existing ulcers.

- Include a structured, comprehensive, and organized educational program as an integral part of quality improvement monitoring. Use information from quality improvement surveys to identify deficiencies, to evaluate the effectiveness of care, and to determine the need for education and policy changes. Focus in-service training on identified deficiencies.

Quality improvement goals help the health care facility or agency provide a program that is comprehensive and consistent with the original program guidelines while having the ability to be monitored, evaluated, and adjusted as patient conditions and current knowledge on pressure ulcer management change. The *AHCPR Clinical Practice Guidelines: Treatment of Pressure Ulcers* recommend the following quality improvement (QI) measures:

- Obtain intradepartmental and interdepartmental QI support for pressure ulcer management as a major aspect of care.

- Convene an interdisciplinary committee of interested and knowledgeable persons to address QI in pressure ulcer management.

- Identify and monitor the occurrence of pressure ulcers to determine their incidence and prevalence. This information serves as a baseline to the development, implementation, and evaluation of treatment protocols.

- Monitor the incidence and prevalence of pressure ulcers on a regular basis.

- Develop, implement, and evaluate educational programs based on the data obtained from QI monitoring.

SUMMARY

The treatment of pressure ulcers should follow the general guidelines and standards of practice for wound management. However, they should also be individualized due to the fact that pressure was the underlying etiology and potentially continues to be a factor in the overall treatment plan. Following the *AHCPR Clinical Practice Guidelines* for treatment of pressure ulcers provides the clinician with a firm, fundamental background upon which to base treatment decisions. The importance of education cannot be emphasized enough in the management of pressure ulcers. Educational programs for patients, caregivers, and health care providers need to be developed. These educational efforts need to target prevention measures as well as treatment measures.

EXAM QUESTIONS

CHAPTER 7
Questions 52-59

52. The two main determinants of pressure ulcer formation are the intensity and duration of pressure and

    a. venous stasis.

    b. nutrition and hydration status of the patient.

    c. tissue tolerance of the skin and supporting structures.

    d. presence of fecal and urinary incontinence.

53. The most common anatomical location for pressure ulcers are the

    a. elbow and occiput.

    b. heel and trochanter.

    c. heel and lateral malleolus.

    d. sacrum and ischium.

54. The percentage of pressure ulcers that develop over the heel is

    a. 8%.

    b. 10%.

    c. 15%.

    d. 20%.

55. The clinical look that shearing pressure ulcers display is

    a. circular.

    b. oval.

    c. triangular.

    d. well demarcated.

56. Moisture adds to the breakdown of intact skin. How many times more likely is moist skin prone to breakdown than is dry skin?

    a. 2 times

    b. 3 times

    c. 4 times

    d. 5 times

57. Full-thickness skin loss involving damage or necrosis of subcutaneous tissue that may extend down to, but not through, underlying fascia is considered a

    a. Stage I pressure ulcer.

    b. Stage II pressure ulcer.

    c. Stage III pressure ulcer.

    d. Stage IV pressure ulcer.

58. An abbreviated nutritional assessment should be performed

    a. monthly.

    b. bimonthly.

    c. every 3 months.

    d. on admission and discharge.

59. The adjunctive therapy for pressure ulcer management that has been endorsed by the *AHCPR Clinical Practice Guidelines: Treatment of Pressure Ulcers* is

    a. electrical stimulation.

    b. growth factors.

    c. hyperbaric oxygen.

    d. ultrasound.

CHAPTER 8

ULCERS OF THE
LOWER EXTREMITIES

CHAPTER OBJECTIVE

Upon completion of the chapter, the reader will distinguish the most common causes of chronic lower leg ulcers and discuss the treatment and teaching related to each etiology.

LEARNING OBJECTIVES

After completion of the chapter, the reader will be able to

1. discuss the etiologies of lower leg ulcers.

2. recognize the assessment characteristics of arterial, venous, and neuropathic ulcers.

3. identify one goal unique to the management of each of the three types of lower leg ulcers.

4. indicate at least two critical items to include in patient education for each of the lower leg ulcers discussed.

INTRODUCTION

Ulcers of the lower extremities are most commonly the result of abnormal circulation. Venous insufficiency causes 75–80% of lower leg ulcers (LLU), and approximately 15–20% of LLUs are a result of arterial insufficiency. Other causes include peripheral neuropathy, vasculitis, various connective tissue disorders, pressure, trauma, pyoderma gangrenosum, malignancy, Raynaud's dis-

ease, necrobiosis lipoidica diabeticorum (NLD), and sickle cell anemia. Ulcers may present with mixed etiologies or coexisting conditions that complicate the healing process.

Comprehensive assessment plays a vital role in identifying predisposing factors and assisting in proper diagnosis (see Table 8-1). The complexity of caring for these ulcerations increases when assessment identifies coexisting pathologies. Identification of underlying etiologies drives treatment decisions and patient management. Treatment needs to include education of the patient and caregiver, not only to ensure consistent treatment but also to prevent recurrence. With proper intervention and teaching, health care providers can make a significant impact on the healing and decreasing recurrence of many LLUs.

VENOUS ULCERS

Venous stasis ulcers are one of the most common vascular disorders (see Figure 8-1). The venous hypertension that results from disorders of the deep venous system eventually gives rise to ulceration. The venous system of the legs consists of three groups of veins: deep veins, superficial veins, and perforator veins. The deep veins are found beneath the fascia and carry the majority of blood out of the legs. The superficial system carries the remainder of the blood and lies within the subcutaneous tissue. The perforator veins connect the deep and superficial sys-

TABLE 8-1 (1 of 2)

Clinical Fact Sheet ◆ QUICK ASSESSMENT OF LEG ULCERS

	VENOUS INSUFFICIENCY (STASIS)	ARTERIAL INSUFFICIENCY	PERIPHERAL NEUROPATHY
HISTORY	◆ Previous DVT and Varicosities ◆ Reduced mobility ◆ Obesity ◆ Vascular Ulcers ◆ Phlebitis ◆ Traumatic Injury ◆ CHF ◆ Orthopedic procedures ◆ Pain reduced by elevation	◆ Diabetes ◆ Anemia ◆ Arthritis ◆ Increased pain with activity and/or elevation ◆ CVA ◆ Smoking ◆ Intermittant claudication ◆ Traumatic injury to extremity ◆ Vascular procedures/surgeries ◆ Hypertension ◆ Hyperlipidemia ◆ Arterial Disease	◆ Diabetes ◆ Spinal Cord injury ◆ Hansens' Disease ◆ Relief of pain with ambulation ◆ Parasthesia of extremities
LOCATION	◆ Medial aspect of lower leg and ankle ◆ Superior to medial malleolus	◆ Toetips or web spaces ◆ Phalangeal heads around lateral malleolus ◆ Areas exposed to pressure or repetitive trauma	◆ Plantar aspect of foot ◆ Metatarsal heads ◆ Heels ◆ Altered pressure points/Sites of Painless Trauma/Repetitive Stress
APPEARANCE	◆ Color: base ruddy ◆ Surrounding skin: erythema (venous dermatitis) and/or brown staining (hyperpigmentation) ◆ Depth: usually shallow ◆ Wound margins: irregular ◆ Exudate: moderate to heavy ◆ Edema: pitting or non-pitting; possible induration and cellulitis ◆ Skin temp: normal; warm to touch ◆ Granulation: frequently present ◆ Infection: less common	◆ Color: base of wound, pale/pallor on elevation; dependent rubor ◆ Skin: shiny, taut, thin, dry, hair loss lower extremities, atrophy of subcutaneous tissue ◆ Depth: deep ◆ Wound margins: even ◆ Exudate: minimal ◆ Edema: variable ◆ Skin temp: decreased/cold ◆ Granulation tissue: rarely present ◆ Infection: frequent (signs may be subtle) ◆ Necrosis, eschar, gangrene may be present	◆ Color: Normal skin tones; trophic skin changes, fissuring and/or callus formation ◆ Depth: variable ◆ Wound margins: well defined ◆ Exudate: variable ◆ Edema: cellulitis, erythema and induration common ◆ Skin temp: warm ◆ Granulation tissue: frequently present ◆ Infection: frequent ◆ Necrotic tissue variable, gangrene uncommon ◆ Reflexes usually diminished ◆ Altered gait; orthopedic deformities common
PERFUSION	**PAIN** ◆ Minimal unless infected or desiccated. **PERIPHERAL PULSES** ◆ Present/Papable **CAPILLARY REFILL** ◆ Normal – less than 3 seconds	**PAIN** ◆ Intermittent claudication ◆ Resting ◆ Positional ◆ Nocturnal **PERIPHERAL PULSES** ◆ Absent or diminished **CAPILLARY REFILL** ◆ Delayed – more than 3 seconds ◆ ABI < 0.8	**PAIN** ◆ Diminished sensitivity to touch ◆ Reduced response to pin prick usually painless **PERIPHERAL PULSES** ◆ Palpable/Present **CAPILLARY REFILL** ◆ Normal

(Continued)

TABLE 8-1 (2 of 2)

Clinical Fact Sheet ◆ QUICK ASSESSMENT OF LEG ULCERS

VENOUS INSUFFICIENCY (STASIS)	ARTERIAL INSUFFICIENCY	PERIPHERAL NEUROPATHY
◆ Measures to improve venous return	◆ Measures to improve tissue perfusion	◆ Measures to eliminate trauma
◆ Surgical obliteration of damaged veins	◆ Revascularization if possible	◆ Pressure relief for heel ulcers
◆ Elevation of legs	◆ Medications to improve RBC transit through narrowed vessels	◆ "Offloading" for plantar ulcers (bedrest **or** contact casting **or** orthopedic shoes)
◆ Compression therapy to provide at least 30mm Hg compression @ ankle	◆ Lifestyle changes (no tobacco, no caffeine, no constrictive garments, avoidance of cold)	◆ Appropriate footwear
Options:	◆ Hydration	◆ Tight glucose control
• Short stretch bandages (e.g. Setopress, Surepress, Comprilan)	◆ Measures to prevent trauma to tissues (appropriate footwear at **all times**)	◆ Aggressive infection control (debridement any necrotic tissue, orthopedic consult for exposed bone, antibiotic coverage)
• Therapeutic support stockings	◆ Topical Therapy	◆ Topical Therapy:
• Unna's Boot	◆ Dry uninfected necrotic wound: keep dry	• Cautious use of occlusive dressings
• Profore 4-layer wrap	◆ Dry infected wound	• Dressing to absorb exudate/keep surface moist
• Compression pumps	◆ Immediate referral for surgical debridement/aggressive antibiotic therapy	
◆ Topical Therapy	◆ Open wound	
◆ Goals: absorb exudate, maintain moist wound surface (e.g. alginate, foam, hydro-colloid dressings)	• Moist wound healing	
	• Nonocclusive dressings (e.g. solid hydrogels) or **cautious** use of occlusive dressings	
	• Aggressive treatment of any infection	

WOCN • 1550 S. Coast Highway, Suite 201 • Laguna Beach, CA 92651 • (888)224-WOCN • Website: http://www.wocn.org

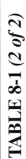

FIGURE 8-1
Venous Ulcer

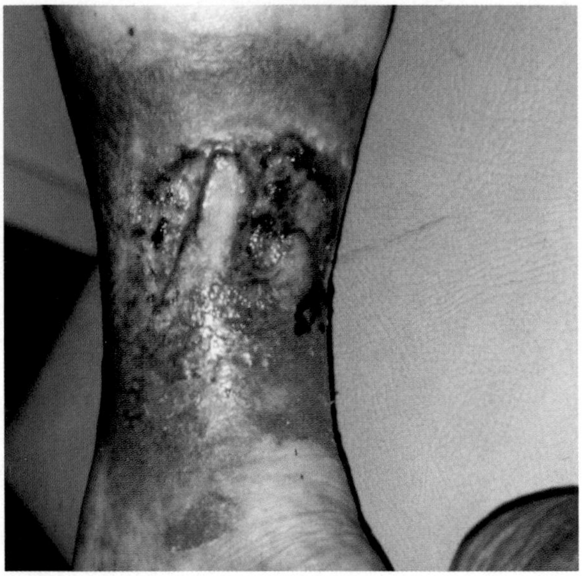

Venous leg ulcer with full-thickness wounds. Note the hemosiderin staining and the irregular wound border.

tems at intervals up the leg. One-way valves are present throughout the veins to prevent backflow and pooling of blood in the leg. The valves keep the flow of blood moving up the leg. The activation of the calf muscle pump occurs with ambulation, assisting with the flow of blood up the leg. Both the one-way valves and the calf muscle pump are necessary to overcome the forces of gravity.

Pooling of blood in the venous system of the legs results from incompetent valves or venous obstruction. When the valves become incompetent, bulging of the veins and backflow of blood occurs. The presence of incompetent valves in the superficial system presents as varicose veins. Numerous disorders are capable of inducing venular dysfunction of the deep system, including thrombosis of the deep venous system, postphlebitic syndrome, congestive heart failure, incompetent valves, obesity, pregnancy, muscle weakness secondary to paralysis, and arthritis. All of these disorders increase venous pressure, resulting in edema and ulceration. The resultant venous hypertension causes increased capillary permeability, leading to leakage, which allows

the passage of erythrocytes, white blood cells, fluid high in protein, and especially fibrinogen, into the surrounding tissue. As metabolic demands for nutrients and oxygen are not met, the cascade of events that follows leads to venous stasis ulceration.

As venous hypertension progresses, the patient presents with lower leg edema, skin changes, and complaints ranging from leg heaviness to leg pain. Generally, skin changes are first seen in the medial gaiter area (medial aspect of the lower leg above the medial malleolus), corresponding to the location of the long saphenous vein of the superficial vein system. The changes begin with erythema, followed by hyperpigmentation. Eventually, classic brawny edema presents as a result of tissue induration and hyperpigmentation. Dryness of the skin promotes pruritus, resulting in skin injury. Weeping from these small breaks in the skin can result when the leg is edematous.

When venous ulcers develop, the wound assessment usually discloses a classic clinical picture. The ulcers are irregular in shape, with ragged borders. The wound base has a beefy red appearance, often with scattered fibrin and moderate to heavy exudate. The extremity is warm and a pulse is present but can be difficult to palpate in the presence of edema. The periulcer skin presents with dermal changes, as previously mentioned. In addition, the skin is often macerated due to excessive exudate. Pain is usually mild.

The primary goal in the treatment of venous ulcers is to focus on the management of edema. Edema is a by-product of poor outflow of blood and the resultant venous hypertension. Wounds do not heal if the edema and underlying venous hypertension are not addressed. Two ways to decrease edema and venous hypertension are to utilize the forces of gravity by elevating the leg and to support the veins to prevent bulging and pooling of blood with the use of compression wraps or support stockings.

An evaluation of arterial flow status is essential to ensure adequate blood flow before any therapeutic support is initiated. As much as 21% of patients with venous ulcers experience concomitant arterial disease. The risk of coexisting arterial dysfunction increases with age (Bryant, 2000). When a patient has both arterial and venous disease, the plan of care becomes complicated (see Figures 8-2 & 8-3). The balance of treating the ulcer and preventing damage is a delicate one, and an inexperienced clinician should seek assistance in managing these situations.

FIGURE 8-2
Mixed Disease Ulcer

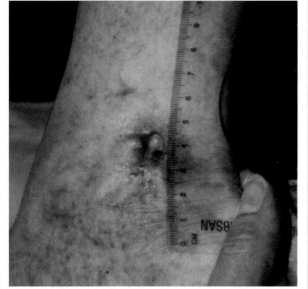

Both arterial and venous insufficiency are present at the malleolus area.

The most common instruction given to the patient is to elevate the legs above the heart. Although this direction is correct, it is sometimes difficult for obese patients or those with respiratory compromise to accomplish adequate elevation. The clinician must work with the patient and caregiver to best accomplish this goal. Remember that because the valves in the veins are incompetent, elevation of the legs has to be high enough to allow a downhill flow.

The recommended compression for venous disease is 30–40 mm Hg. Initially, various compression wraps made for the treatment of venous disease can be used (see Figures 8-4 & 8-5). These wraps give

FIGURE 8-3
Anterior Lower Leg Wound

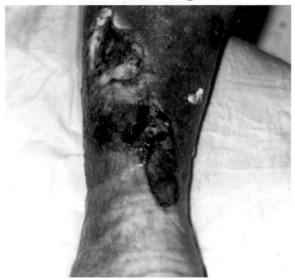

Diabetic patient with venous and arterial insufficiency. Note the necrotic tissue due to ischemia and the hemosiderin staining due to venous hypertension.

sustained, gradual compression over a given time period and have several benefits, including effective accommodation of bulky or absorptive dressings and the enhancement of wound healing by facilitating venous return (thereby managing venous hypertension). Also, by decreasing edema, compression wraps may help to convince the patient that compression is beneficial. Because compression can be uncomfortable for patients, compliance is sometimes an issue.

FIGURE 8-4
Unna's Boot™

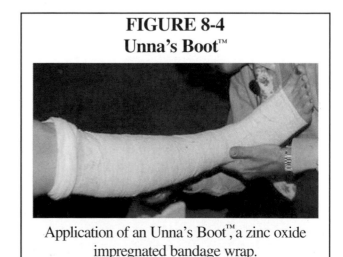

Application of an Unna's Boot™, a zinc oxide impregnated bandage wrap.

FIGURE 8-5
Compression Wraps

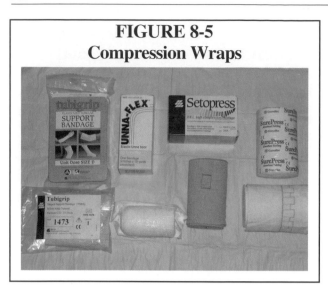

Therapeutic compression stockings can be initiated at any time (see Figure 8-6). Compression is additive, by placing a patient in two 20 mm Hg stockings, one over top of the other, the total compression is 40 mm Hg. This factor is helpful in developing a plan to support the patient in wearing adequate compression. In addition, donning stockings of lesser compression can make the task easier for some patients. Liners are available with only 10 mm Hg compression, which make it easier to get the stockings over dressings and then a 20 or 30 mm Hg stocking can be placed on top to achieve a 30 or 40 mm Hg compression. Several donning tools and devices are also available to assist in getting stockings on, including rubber gloves; fabric assistive devices (see Figure 8-7), and a Donner™ or Butler™, which are similar to a boot pull (see Figure 8-8). Positioning of the stock-

FIGURE 8-6
Compression Stockings

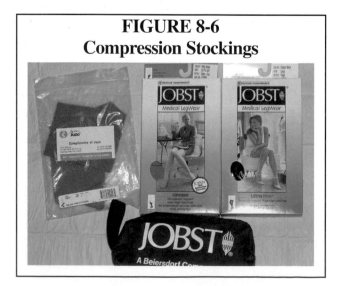

FIGURE 8-7
Donning Tools

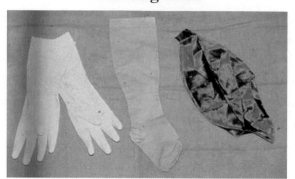

Tools for donning therapeutic stockings (left to right) include dishwashing gloves (also available from stocking manufacturers), therapeutic compression stocking, and slippie (device to don open toe stockings).

FIGURE 8-8
Donning Device

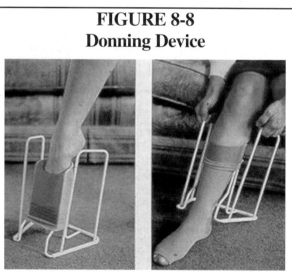

Device used to don therapuetic stockings.

ings before attempting to don, in addition to the position and posture of the patient, can also facilitate application of compression stockings.

The use of therapeutic support stockings is essential and should be introduced as soon as possible in the treatment plan. Their use is of utmost importance not only in the treatment of venous ulcers but in the prevention of their recurrence as well. Convincing the patient that the benefits of support stockings outweigh the detriments can be a challenge. Support stockings are difficult to don, are hot in summer weather, and are expensive. The commitment to wear support stockings must be life-long, however, this commitment is not only a compliance issue but also a financial one. Because, support stockings must be replaced every 4–6 months to ensure adequate compression therapy, they can be quite costly. The clinician also needs to ensure that the patient has properly fitting stockings; often patients purchase a larger size because they are not as tight and therefore, easier to don. A trained fitter, usually at a durable medical supply company, is invaluable.

Effective October 1, 2003, Medicare beneficiaries with venous insufficiency and open wounds are eligible for coverage for support stockings. Unfortunately, no Medicare coverage exists for prevention before or after ulceration; however, professional organizations, such as the Wound, Ostomy, and Continence Nurses Society, continue to work on legislative changes. Some state Medicaid programs (for example, California's MediCal) cover stockings for the diagnosis of chronic venous insufficiency and can therefore be used even after healing to prevent recurrence or new ulceration. Well-fitting compression stockings, along with continued education and regular checkups, are the basis for preventing recurrences (Poore, Cameron, & Cherry, 2002).

As with any wound, the topical treatment of a venous wound follows moist wound healing principles to promote wound repair. The theory behind moist wound healing and a description of types of wound products appear in chapter 9. The challenge to the provider is management of the sometimes excessive exudate. The goal of maintaining a moist wound bed and dry intact skin directs choices through the course of treatment. The frequency of dressing changes to manage exudate and the ability of the patient to don therapeutic support stockings or tolerate various compression amounts influences the provider's choice of treatment. The plan of care needs frequent reevaluation as the wound progresses toward healing.

ARTERIAL ULCERS

Lower-extremity arterial disease is the inadequate supply of blood to the tissues and skin of the foot and leg. Arterial blood flow is essential to the delivery of nutrients and oxygen at the cellular level. When the oxygen requirement rises, blood flow cannot increase to meet this demand, and an ischemic environment results. When peripheral arterial occlusion becomes severe, the mechanism of peripheral vasodilation is inadequate to meet the needs of skin, muscle, and nerves, even at rest (Bonham & Flemister, 2002). This condition is commonly associated with the term *peripheral vascular disease* (PVD), which literally includes conditions involving all of the peripheral vessels: the arteries, veins, and lymphatics. The more accurate term for this condition is lower-extremity arterial disease (LEAD).

Atherosclerosis is the most common cause of LEAD. Identified risk factors for LEAD include the use of tobacco products, advanced age, hyperlipidemia, diabetes mellitus, hypertension, obesity, and a family history of cardiovascular disease (Bonham & Flemister, 2002). Atherosclerotic changes of the arteries occur as a result of plaque formation. This process is promoted by smoking and diabetes mellitus.

Leg pain caused by ischemia is a classic sign of arterial insufficiency. Usually first evident as intermittent claudication, the pain is proportional to the ischemia. As the ischemic condition progresses, pain increases. At rest, a patient can tolerate up to a 70% occlusion of an artery; however, with exercise, the increased circulation demands cannot be met, and muscle ischemia results in crampy leg pain. Rest pain occurs when a 90% or greater occlusion exists (Bryant, 2000). Exercise can increase collateral circulation and, thereby, slowly increase the distance the patient can walk before symptoms of ischemic pain occur.

The characteristics most commonly associated with arterial ulcers include well-demarcated wound margins; a painful, deep, often full-thickness wound; and a wound bed with either nonviable gray-yellow tissue or eschar or, if the wound bed is clean, pale coloration due to compromised blood flow (see Figures 8-9 & 8-10). Because of the ischemic condition, signs of the inflammatory response are muted and cellulitis is often subtle. Typical locations for arterial ulcers include the ankles and feet; the lateral malleoli especially; the toes or tips of toes, over phalangeal heads; and areas of trauma. When arterial insufficiency occurs, the limb is pale and cool, and has poor capillary refill and evidence of hair loss is present.

FIGURE 8-9
Arterial Ulcer

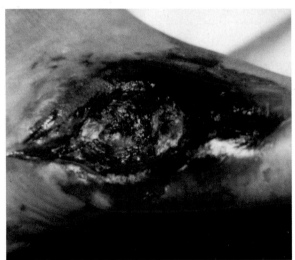

Arterial ulcer on the lateral aspect of the foot. Significant arterial insufficiency is present with acute infection.

FIGURE 8-10
Diabetic Ulcers

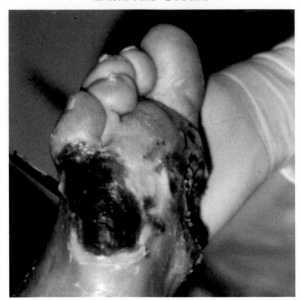

Diabetic peripheral neuropathy with arterial insufficiency.

Assessment of the affected extremity identifies six typical characteristics. These characteristics are commonly referred to as the six Ps of arterial insufficiency

- Pain
- Pallor
- Pulselessness
- Polar (cold)
- Paresthesia
- Paralysis.

The clinician has to consider the coexistence of other disease processes that can mask these signs. For example, if coexisting peripheral neuropathy or paresthesia is present, the symptom of pain may be absent. When venous disease exists, the color of the extremity may resemble the brown discoloration seen with venous insufficiency (as seen in Figure 8-3).

Patients with arterial disease require assessment of arterial flow. Vascular studies, both noninvasive and invasive, are performed to determine the extent of disease and potential for surgical revascularization. Noninvasive tests include ankle brachial index

(ABI), toe pressures, transcutaneous oxygen tension, and duplex scanning. Angiography is an invasive test used to visualize the vascular system.

Management of the patient with an arterial ulcer is often complex because of coexisting morbidities. A multidisciplinary team approach is essential in treating coexisting medical conditions, healing the ulcer, and minimizing recurrence. A comprehensive management plan must initially evaluate the cause of the arterial ulcer. Because it is ischemic in nature, measures to improve perfusion, including the use of pharmacological agents and the building of collateral circulation and revascularization, are considered. Factors contributing to the decreased perfusion or local cause of the arterial ulcer — including smoking; repetitive trauma, such as improper shoe wear; dehydration; and constrictive clothing or socks, which may impede blood flow and enhance edema — must also be eliminated. In effort to decrease pain, the patient may dangle the leg over the side of the bed at night or sleep sitting up in a chair. With the help of gravity, blood flow is enhanced, and pain is relieved. However, edema often occurs due to the dependent position of the extremity. Addressing these factors is critical in the overall management of the wound.

Before decisions about local care can be undertaken, several considerations need to be addressed. Foremost, what is the degree of circulation? Is there enough blood flow available to heal the wound? Blood is needed to control the level of bacteria in the wound, rid the wound of necrotic tissue, and produce granulation tissue to heal the wound. Local wound care is based on the principles covered in the "Moist Wound Healing" section of chapter 10. The treatment for arterial ulcers varies depending upon the presence or absence of adequate blood supply. Debridement is the treatment of choice for non ischemic wounds. However, debridement is contraindicated in the presence of dry gangrene or a stable, dry ischemic wound. Once an ischemic wound with eschar develops odor, erythema, or drainage, then the clinician must reevaluate treatment and the need for debridement. Tissue loss can be minimized if vascular supply is restored. This allows the wound to demarcate or for self-amputation to occur; otherwise, appropriate amputation procedures may need to be performed (Bryant, 2000).

The presence of infection must be continually evaluated. When drainage or pain increases in an arterial ulcer, the clinician should suspect infection, and cultures are indicated. Osteomyelitis is a concern when an ulcer lies over a bony prominence, especially when the ulcer is chronic. A significant number of patients have both arterial disease and diabetes. These patients are at high risk for the development of peripheral neuropathy, which masks the signs of infection and decreases the response to repetitive trauma.

In addition to ulcer management, the patient needs to understand how lifestyle choices affect the disease process. The slow progression of an arterial ulcer occurs as the already diminshed blood flow is inadequate to meet the additional demands created by the ulcer. There are several measures a patient can take to minimize vasoconstriction and help maximize the blood flow. Cold temperatures should be avoided by keeping the room warm and wearing cotton or wool socks. All efforts to stop smoking should be made due to the detrimental effects on the arterioles. The patient should also avoid wearing constrictive socks. Trauma to the lower extremities should also be avoided. Diabetic footcare guidelines are appropriate for patients with arterial insufficiency. Light exercise and activity can assist with developing collateral circulation in arterial insufficiency but must be limited when an ulcer is present. Remember the demand of blood flow increases in an attempt to heal the ulcer. The patient can particiapte in their care by performing these measures.

Arterial ulcers are usually chronic in nature, and PVD is a progressive disease. There is no cure for PVD. Treatment aims to control the disease and curtail complications.

NEUROPATHIC ULCERS

Neuropathic ulcers have long been associated with diabetic neuropathy and, therefore, may be referred to as diabetic foot ulcers. Actually, however peripheral neuropathy can accompany myriad diseases, including Hansen's disease, alcoholism, vitamin deficiencies, collagen disease, herniated disc, uremia, pernicious anemia, and untoward effects of pharmacological agents. This discussion focuses on diabetic neuropathy, because it is the most common of the peripheral neuropathies.

The pathophysiology of peripheral neuropathy in a patient with diabetes is a complex cascade of events. It is multifactorial, with hyperglycemia playing a prominent, but not sole, role (Bryant, 2000). Sensory neuropathy (diminished or lossed sensation that leads to the "insensate foot") has been the main focus of diabetic neuropathy. The motor and autonomic components of neuropathy have been largely ignored despite their profound influence on the lower extremities. Each plays a role in the development of neuropathic ulceration, a true pressure ulcer. The most common causes of neuropathic ulcers are pressure and traumatic injury.

Sensory neuropathy causes altered sensation. Sometimes this altered sensation is manifested as hypersensitivity, but more commonly it appears as diminished or lack of sensation; loss of proprioception; and loss of temperature sensation. Consequently, painless trauma occurs, leading to ulceration. This is usually bilateral and symmetrical, occurring distally first and ascending as the process continues. In motor neuropathy, the intrinsic muscles of the foot are initially affected, permitting digital contractures (Kominsky, 1994). Autonomic neuropathy accounts for the excessive dryness of the skin that leads to cracking and fissuring, making the foot more prone to infection (see Figure 8-11).

FIGURE 8-11
Toes

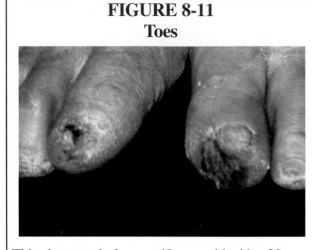

This photograph shows a 40-year-old with a 20-year history of diabetes, not well controlled. Fissures in the foot, heels, and toes, most likely resulting from autonomic peripheral neuropathy, have occurred. These fissures can be open to bacteria.

Foot deformities and neuropathies need to be included in the clinical assessment. When foot deformities occur, pressure points on the foot change, the normal gait is altered, and commonly the foot is insensate, leading to poor outcomes. Early screening and intervention can prevent most neuropathic ulcer development. Plantar ulcers develop over areas of highest pressure (Birke, Pavich, Patout, & Horswell, 2002). Common sites are the first and third metatarsal heads; when Charcot's foot is present, the midfoot is a high-risk site. The increase in pressure is a result of the structural bone changes (see Figure 8-12). Each clinician should employ off-loading of the area. Off-loading is used to disperse the pressure on the plantar surface or walking surface of the foot, eliminating high pressure over the area of concern. Many temporary and permanent options are available, including non-weight bearing, total contact cast, shoe inserts, wide-depth shoes, custom shoes, pneumatic walkers, and accommodative felt and foam dressings. A total contact cast is considered the gold standard (Birke et al., 2002) because it results in reduction of vertical pressure at the pressure points of the foot and reduction of shearing forces by immobilizing the foot and permitting ambulation. Keep in mind that neuropathic ulcers are pressure ulcers, therefore, the contributing factor, pressure, must be eliminated. The risks and benefits of each method are not in the scope of this discussion but it is imperative that each clinician develop a system or resource to supplement their treatment plan. Off-loading is needed not only in the treatment of neuropathic ulcers but also in prevention. The clinician should consult a podiatrist or orthotist for advice on off-loading techniques. Once again, patient education is imperative. Unless patients are first convinced of the importance of and become dedicated to the commitment of off-loading, daily foot care, and prevention, any wound care the clinician initiates becomes ineffective.

nosis; common sites for neuropathic ulcer development are areas that receive trauma and pressure. Walking can even cause areas of pressure. Common sites are the plantar aspect of the foot, the overlying metatarsal heads, the area under the heel, the plantar aspect of the great toe, and the tops of the toes. Areas of callus represent areas of pressure, whether around an existing wound or on another area of the foot. A callus is a warning sign to relieve pressure. The presence of a callus, in and of itself, increases pressure to the underlying tissues. Polymicrobial cellulitis and osteomyelitis are prevalent with neuropathic ulcers. The clinician must also assess for coexisting arterial disease.

FIGURE 8-12
Neuropathic Foot Ulcer

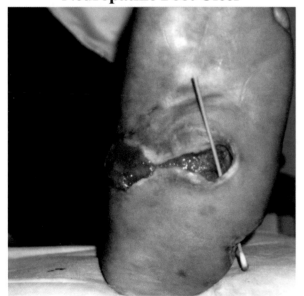

New pressure points develop as a result of Charcot's foot deformity in this diabetic patient with peripheral neuropathy.

FIGURE 8-13
Diabetic Foot Ulcers

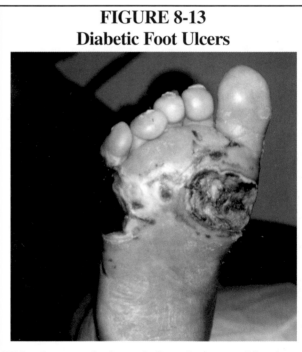

This photograph shows infected neuropathic ulcers with arterial insufficiency. Medial wound status post debridement with lateral wound eschar.

A neuropathic ulcer has distinctive characteristics: it usually has painless, even wound margins; callused edges and surrounding skin caused by continued pressure; and a deep, red, granular base. If arterial insufficiency is also present, the wound bed will be pale or necrotic (see Figure 8-13). Pulses should be present on a neuropathic limb unless arterial disease is present. Location also assists in diag-

It is a common myth that diabetic ulcers do not heal. A true, or pure, neuropathic ulcer has a good blood supply and has the ability to heal with appropriate wound care, aggressive off loading, and controlled blood sugars. If no coexisting arterial insufficiency exists, then the blood supply is available and the etiology of pressure must be addressed. Local care is based on moist wound healing (see chapter 10) and aggressive debridement, which has been shown to improve healing rates. These measures, along off-loading, are necessary to reach the goal of a healed ulcer. Success in decreasing recurrence as well as healing of current ulcers depends largely on patient education. Patients must understand the importance of preventive care so as to decrease their financial burden and more importantly to take care of their feet. Teaching must be comprehensive. The patient must understand the risks and be willing to comply with the treatment regimen. A patient who states willingness to stay off of the ulcer but arrives at every clinic visit walking needs further education to encourage compliance with the whole treatment plan.

A team approach is critical in the management of the diabetic neuropathic limb. It is well documented that the prevention of diabetic foot complications requires the involvement of multiple disciplines in care (Bowker & Pfeifer, 2001). The following foot care instructions for the patient with diabetes need to be included in any plan of care

- Careful daily inspection of the feet for blisters, scratches, and red areas needs to be carried out. If the patient's vision is impaired, another person needs to do the inspection.

- Wash the patient's feet daily in warm water and dry carefully between the toes.

- Remember that a neuropathic foot has loss of temperature sensation and, therefore, cannot adequately gauge water temperature; bath water must always be tested prior to the patient entering it.

- Avoid corn removal using "bathroom surgery" or application of strong chemicals; have the patient see a podiatrist regularly.

- Ensure that properly fitting shoes are worn. New shoes should be worn for short intermittent intervals only and foot inspection should be performed upon shoe removal.

- Tell the patient not to wear open-toed shoes and sandals or walk barefoot, due to the risk of trauma.

Instruction is the easy part. The difficult task is convincing the patient how important foot care is in the prevention of ulceration and limb salvage.

SUMMARY

Ulcerations in the lower leg can result from venous insufficiency, arterial ischemia, or peripheral neuropathy. To enhance healing, maximize efforts, and prevent recurrence, follow specific management principles for each of the underlying etiologies. Patient education plays a key role in the success of ulcer prevention for each type, especially venous and neuropathic ulcers. The complexity of management is further complicated when mixed etiologes are present. The mixtures are commonly neuropathy and arterial disease or venous and arterial disease. A multidisciplinary approach is critical for successful patient care management.

CASE STUDY

Mr. Walker*, a 52-year-old male patient, presented to the wound clinic with a chronic lower leg ulcer. The ulcer has been present for 4 years and Mr. Walker is now on disability. He was unable to walk and stand at his job because of pain at the wound site and a large amount of drainage. He came to the clinic with an Unna's Boot,™ which he changed once a week.

On the first visit, he would not allow anyone to remove the dressing due to pain and removed it himself. Mr. Walker was distrustful of staff members; he had seen many clinicians in the past 4 years. We assessed the ulcer and arterial circulation (see Figure 8-14). An Unna's Boot™ was reapplied and instruction was given to change it two times per week and to use a zinc oxide-based moisture barrier around the wound. The wound bed had more than 50% scattered slough, the periwound skin was macerated, the wound was painful, and the leg had 2+ pitting edema. We were unable to change any other

*Name has been changed to protect patient confidentiality.

FIGURE 8-14
Lower Leg Ulcer

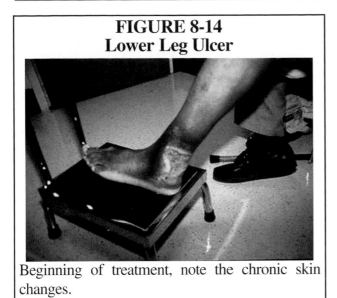

Beginning of treatment, note the chronic skin changes.

aspect of his care, so we took the opportunity to teach him about venous disease. We stressed the need to increase venous return through elevation and compression. He agreed to elevate his leg and change the Unna's Boot™ twice a week.

On the second and third weekly visit, the edema decreased and the maceration improved (see Figure 8-15). The pain was slowly decreasing, and Mr. Walker saw a slight improvement with the increased dressing change. We were able to place more absorptive dressings, using a calcium alginate and foam under a four-layer bandage. This allowed for more control of the exudate, keeping it contained over the wound and off the periwound skin. The four-layer bandage system delivered sustained compression

FIGURE 8-15
Lower Leg Ulcer

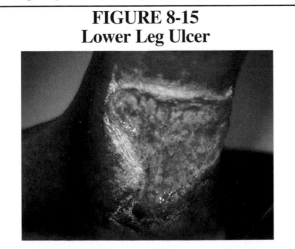

Wound bed early in treatment; note the protection to the periwound skin from the excessive drainage.

over the week of approximately 40 mm Hg. Mr. Walker was more receptive to listening about the benefits and types of compression. We had already introduced the idea of therapeutic stockings.

Subsequent visits continued to show improvement. As we gained the patient's trust, the wound improved and the pain was eliminated (see Figure 8-16). Gradually, the calcium alginate was discontinued and only the foam was needed to contain the exudate for the week. We continued with the four-layer wrap. The patient was receptive to teaching and began to perform ankle and foot exercises in addition to increasing the amount of walking per week.

FIGURE 8-16
Lower Leg Ulcer

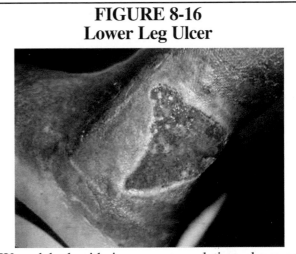

Wound bed with increase granulation, decrease edema and improvement of periwound skin as exudate is controlled.

The day came that the wound was clearly on the way to healing. The patient finally agreed to therapeutic compression stockings to allow for daily showering, dressing changes, and less frequent office visits (see Figure 8-17). The patient was faithful to wearing the stockings and much happier, greatly improving his quality of life.

As a follow-up note, the patient changed to another insurance but did heal shortly after he left our clinic. About 1 year later, Mr. Walker came by to visit the clinic. He informed us that his ulcer had reoccurred. Upon further questioning, the patient admitted to not wearing his stockings regularly for

FIGURE 8-17
Lower Leg Ulcer

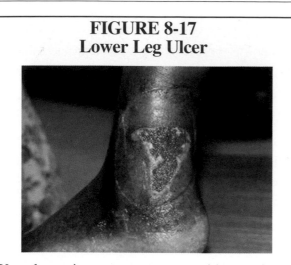

Wound continues to progress with consistent compression.

about 3–4 months. He told us that his current health care provider had told him that when the ulcer healed, he could return to his stockings; at that time, there was no compression.

We asked the patient how he thought the ulcer would heal without the underlying etiology being addressed. We had a long discussion with the patient about what we had taught him. The patient understood what the problem was, he just needed reminding and reinforcement of teaching. It was up to him to decide what to do; unfortunately, his present providers were not treating him according to the standards of care for venous insufficiency with ulceration. The patient was never seen again, but I believe he thought about how the first ulcer had healed and probably became more active in his care. Once again, patient education is paramount in healing wounds. Education is imperative for patients and their families to continue the lifelong commitment of the prevention plan. Clinical providers must also understand the pathophysiology of the disease to initiate treatment plans that target the etiology.

EXAM QUESTIONS

CHAPTER 8
Questions 60-72

60. Abnormal leg circulation that results in pooling of blood and leakage of fluid into the interstitial tissue is

    a. arterial insufficiency.
    b. Raynaud's disease.
    c. venous insufficiency.
    d. peripheral neuropathy.

61. The primary goal in the treatment of venous ulcers is to focus on the management of

    a. edema.
    b. exudate.
    c. pain.
    d. veins.

62. Characteristics of a leg assessment for venous ulceration may reveal

    a. pulse, cool extremity, loss of hair, and hyperpigmentation in gaiter area.
    b. pulse, brawny edema, irregular wound edges, and excessive exudate.
    c. absent pulse, brawny edema, red granular wound bed, and insensate foot.
    d. brawny edema, well-defined wound margins, and dry wound bed.

63. The length of time that compression therapy must be used for chronic venous insufficiency is

    a. until the ulcer is healed.
    b. until the edema is well controlled.
    c. lifelong.
    d. 4–6 months.

64. Before beginning compression therapy for venous ulceration, the clinician must

    a. have a vascular consult.
    b. wait until the ulcer has healed by 75%.
    c. establish the presence of adequate blood flow.
    d. test the patient's blood sugar.

65. The symptom that indicates a 90% or greater arterial occlusion is

    a. intermittent claudication.
    b. pale wound bed.
    c. infection.
    d. rest pain.

66. The six Ps of arterial insufficiency are

    a. pain, pallor, pulse, polar, paresthesia, and paralysis.
    b. pain, pallor, pulselessness, polar, pressure, and paralysis.
    c. pain, pallor, pulselessness, polar, paresthesia, and paralysis.
    d. painless, pallor, pulse, polar, paresthesia, and paralysis.

67. The local care treatment option that is contraindicated for a dry, stable, ischemic arterial ulcer is

    a. pressure relief.

    b. dry gauze dressing.

    c. amputation.

    d. debridement.

68. The complications of infection and osteomyelitis are more prevalent in

    a. venous stasis ulcer.

    b. neuropathic ulcer.

    c. full-thickness granulating wound.

    d. partial-thickness wound.

69. The most common causes of neuropathic ulcers are

    a. pressure and traumatic injury.

    b. pressure and arterial insufficiency.

    c. infection and osteomyelitis.

    d. traumatic injury and arterial insufficiency.

70. In peripheral neuropathy, excessive dry skin with resultant fissures is a result of

    a. sensory neuropathy.

    b. motor neuropathy.

    c. autonomic neuropathy.

    d. arterial neuropathy.

71. For a patient with a neuropathic ulcer, an important teaching point is for the patient to

    a. wear open-toed shoes.

    b. perform bathroom surgery.

    c. use over-the-counter chemicals to reduce calluses or corns.

    d. avoid weight bearing on the ulcer.

72. Callus formation is most commonly associated with

    a. continued pressure.

    b. chronicity of a wound.

    c. infection.

    d. macerated skin.

CHAPTER 9

MANAGING WOUNDS WITH EDEMA

CHAPTER OBJECTIVES

After completion of this chapter, the reader will have an understanding of the differences between generalized edema and lymphedema, formation of lymphedema, classifications and stages of lymphedema, cornerstone of therapy for lymphedema, and effect of edema on wound management. The reader will also be able to recognize and formulate important aspects of edema management and be aware of the referral process.

LEARNING OBJECTIVES

After completion of this chapter, the reader will be able to

1. state how generalized edema and lymphedema are formed.

2. name the classifications and stages of lymphedema.

3. indicate three characteristics of lymphedema.

4. describe the main treatment options for edema and lymphedema.

INTRODUCTION

The presence of edema can make the management of medical conditions more difficult, and it certainly adds another component when managing wound care. The etiologies of edema may be related to a long-standing disease process or may be acute, such as with trauma. Edema may also be associated with the lymphatic system (lymphedema). One of the wound care goals for complications associated with edema is to reduce the edema and allow for optimal healing to take place. General options for edema reduction have always included elevation and compression; however, additional treatment methods or referrals are also now available for general edema and lymphedema management. This chapter provides information on the management of edema with wound care.

GENERALIZED EDEMA

Wounds tend to heal slower or not at all in an environment that has an edema component. Edema, or swelling, interferes with the usual vascular flow of oxygen and cellular nutrients that are needed for wound repair. Edema secondary to surgery or trauma is a natural response by the body to this type of injury. Water and body fluids without high levels of protein usually comprise this type of edema. Treatment with elevation, ice, anti-inflammatory medications, diuretics, or compression therapy usually assists in improvement of edema. Leg elevation of 18 cm above the heart level for 2–4 hours each day has been found to be an effective regimen. If the lower extremities are elevated above the heart level for more prolonged periods, edema is reduced even more, improving microcirculation, especially for patients with venous insufficiency (Hess, 2002; Milne, Corbett, & Dubuc, 2003).

Lower extremity edema is commonly seen in venous disease due to elevated venous pressure that pushes fluids through distended and permeable capillary beds into the surrounding tissues. Acute onset of lower extremity edema is associated with etiologies such as deep vein thrombosis (DVT), cellulitis, surgery, and trauma. Chronic edema with venous insufficiency has more of a gradual onset with an increase in edema with dependent positions and a decrease in edema with elevation (see Figure 9-1) (Bryant, 2000).

FIGURE 9-1
Venous Insufficiency

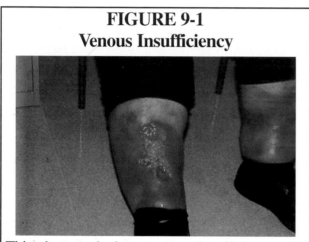

This photograph shows venous insufficiency with ulcerations. Once edema was controlled, these ulcers healed. A four-layer wrap was used for several weeks; then therapeutic compression stockings were worn all day by this male patient. The patient continued to work throughout treatment but remained faithful about wearing his stockings.

Whatever the reason for edema, the wound healing process is usually affected. Edema can increase the force on injured tissue and compromise blood flow, rendering the physiologic effects of the inflammatory phase less effective. Excessive swelling can result in nerve compression, which may increase pain and further decrease blood flow. This is seen and most evident in compartment syndrome (Milne, Corbett, & Dubuc, 2003).

Third space or interstitial fluid collection mechanically compromises the microvascular and lymphatic system, which results in a decrease in the delivery of oxygen and nutrients to the tissues and a decrease in the removal of wound healing inhibitory factors and toxins. It has been shown in cases with chronic venous insufficiency that when lymphedema was removed, a significant increase in transcutaneous oxygen tension occurs. In-vitro studies have shown that fluids removed from chronic wounds suppressed the proliferation of keratinocytes, fibroblasts, and vascular endothelial cells (MacDonald, 2001).

LYMPHEDEMA

Lymphedema can be a significant detriment to wound management as well as to the long-term planning and prevention of future wound and skin irritation. Lymphedema is not as common as edema from chronic venous insufficiency or generalized edema from surgery, trauma, or similar etiologies, but it has been estimated to affect approximately 1 person in 30 throughout the world (MacDonald, 2001). The importance of understanding its management, however, is extremely valuable in order to obtain the best patient outcomes with appropriate treatment.

The origin of lymphedema is the lymphatic system. The lymphatic system works in conjunction with the vascular system to maintain a normal plasma volume. The protein-rich fluid from the vascular system that moves out of the bloodstream into the interstitial space is not completely returned to the bloodstream. The high-protein fluid that remains in the interstitial space is picked up by the lymphatic system. Eventually, this fluid is returned to the vascular flow, making the lymphatic system an important player in normal plasma volume. The lymphatic system also assists in removing toxic substances and damaged cells from the tissues, defending against malignancy, and protecting against infections by way of lymph tissue and nodes. Several lymph nodes are positioned at various points along the larger lymphatic channels. These nodes contain lymphocytes, which assist in clearing the lymph drainage of toxic substances and pathogens harmful to the human body (Bryant, 2000).

Lymphedema occurs when the protein-rich fluid of the lymphatic system collects abnormally in the tissues as a result of either an increase in the amount of lymph produced or a compromise in the lymph drainage system. The composition of this fluid, with its plasma proteins, attracts additional water, leading to increased swelling. Lymphedema can be classified as either primary or secondary. Primary lymphedema is a more rare, inherited form in which the lymph nodes and vessels are either absent or abnormal. This type of edema accounts for about 10% of the cases of lymphedema. Secondary lymphedema occurs when the lymphatic system is blocked or disrupted (see Figures 9-2 and 9-3). Common causes of secondary lymphedema include radiation therapy, trauma, cancer, surgery involving the lymph nodes, infection, filariasis, venous disease, and obesity. Secondary lymphedema may be seen immediately after surgery or it may be absent for many years (MacDonald, 2001; Milne, Corbett, & Dubuc, 2003).

FIGURE 9-2
Lymphedema

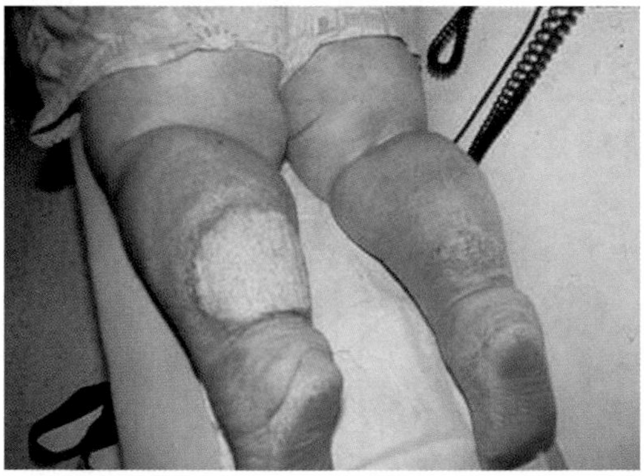

Lymphedema following a bug bite several years before.

FIGURE 9-3
Close-up of Lymphedema

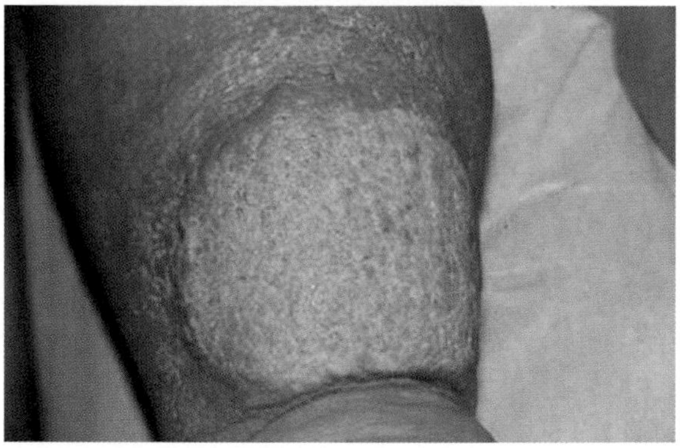

Close-up of the left leg wound from lymphedema in Figure 9-2.

There are three stages of lymphedema. Stage I is described as edema that comes and goes without any particular treatment. Stage II lymphedema is characterized by pitting of the tissues that underlie the epidermis. The pitting appearance can take up to 15 minutes to dissipate after the tissues have been depressed. Stage III lymphedema is characterized by chronic skin changes and is described as having an orange-peel appearance with a hard, wood-like feeling (termed indurosis). Indurosis is commonly seen with both stage II and stage III lymphedema. Fibrosis, on the otherhand, describes irreversible hardening of tissue that is usually soft. This characteristic is seen quite often with chronic venous insufficiency of the lower legs (Milne, Corbett, & Dubuc, 2003).

Lymphedema usually manifests itself as a progressive edema that begins in the distal-most portion of the extremity, either the hand or the foot, and moves upward. The edema often produces a hump on the dorsal portion of the foot. Toe involvement is also common. As the edema worsens, and the lymph fluid continues to accumulate in the tissues, a severe distortion of the limb can be noted with destruction of the elastic components of the skin. This condition is referred to as elephantiasis. The protein deposits in the skin cause progressive thickening and fibrosis of the skin. The compromised lymphatic system is a concern for the clinician because the system is much less able to manage any bacterial challenge. Very small breaks in the skin may lead to acute cellulitis. Any trauma or infectious process that affects the location of the lymphedema provides additional inflammation and fibrosis, which cascades into further damage of the compromised lymphatic system (Bryant, 2000).

Lymphedema may be diagnosed through family history, medical history, lymphoscintigraphy, or lymphangiography. The family history may show a genetic component that would indicate primary lymphedema. Medical or surgical history may describe removal of lymph nodes or trauma that would disrupt the lymph system, leading to secondary lymphedema. Lymphoscintigraphy and lymphangiography are X-ray procedures in which the lymphatic system and the lymph nodes are visualized after a contrast medium is injected. External evaluation by physical examination can lead to additional findings that assist in the diagnosis of lymphedema. Palpation of the edematous area and evaluation of the skin's color, temperature, turgor, and texture help with the diagnosis of fibrosis or indurosis. Evaluation of any drainage or weeping areas must be addressed in the plan of treatment (Milne, Corbett, & Dubuc, 2003).

TREATMENT OF GENERALIZED EDEMA AND LYMPHEDEMA

As mentioned, treatment for generalized edema includes elevation, ice, anti-inflammatory medications, diuretics, and compression therapy. These methods usually improve the edema, especially when it is of rapid onset from an etiology such as surgery or trauma. Elevation needs to be high enough — 18 cm above heart level has been found to be adequate to decrease edema. For chronic venous insufficiency and venous stasis ulcers, compression therapy is the mainstay of treatment (see Figure 9-4). Compression therapy was covered in greater detail in chapter 8,

specifically in relation to lower extremity ulcers; however, a variety of compression methods are available, from elastic wraps to compression hose and pneumatic pumps. Management of chronic edema from venous insufficiency requires a long-term plan of care that the patient believes in and will be consistent with in its implementation (Hess, 2002; Milne, Corbett, & Dubuc, 2003).

FIGURE 9-4
Venous Disease

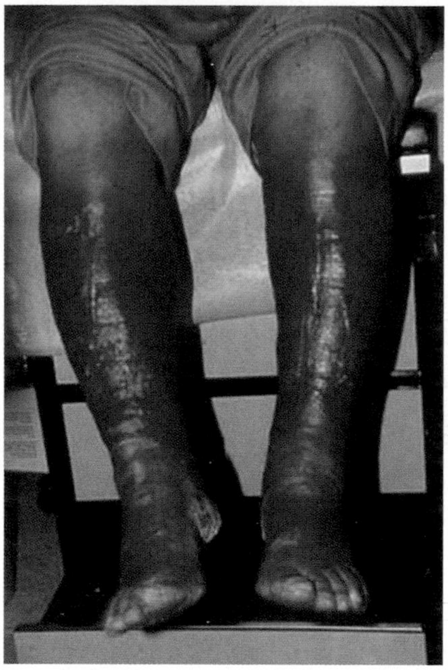

This photograph shows a male patient with venous disease and scattered small ulcerations. This patient worked standing on his feet all day. We successfully treated him while he continued to work. Note the decreasing edema achieved through compression wraps.

Management of lymphedema is focused on the mobilization of lymph fluid, with reduction of edema and restoration of the usual limb contours, maintenance of the restored state of edema reduction, and prevention of infection. Therapy can be divided into two main categories: restorative (also referred to as volumetric reduction) and maintenance (Bryant, 2000).

The mainstay of therapy for lymphedema is comprehensive decongestive physiotherapy (CDP). This therapy is comprised of manual lymph drainage, compression bandaging, patient education that includes prevention and self-care, and exercises. Understanding how compression bandaging works with lymphedema is essential for the clinician. Low-stretch bandaging is used in the management of lymphedema. Low-stretch bandages have a high "working pressure" and a low "resting pressure." What this means to the patient with lymphedema is that when the patient is relaxed and not moving, the bandages supply a comfortable level of support that is tolerable to wear on a long-term basis. When the patient walks or exercises, the "working pressure" increases as the muscles contract against the fixed resistance of the bandages, causing an effective, intermittent massage on the tissues that forces lymphatic fluid from the interstitial spaces into the lymphatic collectors. These functioning collectors mobilize the lymphatic fluid for removal, with the end results being decreased edema and a more functional limb. As for any patient with ischemia or an insensate limb, special precautions must be used to evaluate the use of compression bandaging or stockings. (Chapter 8 discusses this in more detail.) Elevation of the involved limb is also helpful. Diuretics are rarely indicated with lymphedema unless there is a significant amount of generalized edema in addition to the underlying lymphedema, such as is seen with congestive heart failure (MacDonald, 2001).

Treatment components for lymphedema, which are related to the restorative or mobilization phase of edema, are CDP, sequential compression therapy, limb elevation, and compression bandaging.

- CDP involves the use of therapeutic massage to mobilize lymph fluid, followed by use of compression bandages. The massage therapy is performed by therapists who have been trained in this specialized technique. Massage therapy involves 1–2 sessions daily for 1–3 weeks.

- Sequential compression pumps have limb sleeves that are applied to the affected areas and,

when inflated, compress the lymphatics, which increases the lymph flow. Once again, after treatment, compression wraps or garments are used to keep the fluid from returning to the interstitial spaces.

- Limb elevation decreases edema by countering the effects of gravity on the lymphatic flow. Elevation is most effective in the early stages of lymphedema.

The maintenance phase of lymphedema management also relies heavily on compression bandaging and custom stockings or sleeves, as well as patient exercises and skin and nail care.

- Compression bandaging is not only used to mobilize the fluid on initial treatment but is a mainstay of long-term therapy. Short-stretch or inelastic bandages and custom measured sleeves and stockings are the most effective types of compression therapies. The compression bandages apply pressure to the tissues, which compresses the lymphatics, and move the lymph fluid in the interstitial spaces into the lymphatic channels.

- Patient exercises assist in the maintenance of lymph reduction. The exercises stimulate the intact lymphatic system and increase the rate of lymphatic transport, which improves the general mobilization of the fluid. The exercises are taught by a therapist, and patients are instructed to exercise with compression garments or bandages in place.

- Skin and nail care is extremely important in the prevention of infection and in long-term maintenance. Excellent skin and nail care helps to keep the skin supple and prevents many of the breaks in the skin that can be caused by minor trauma or dry skin. Prevention measures decrease the likelihood of infection. Nail care assists in the reduction of minor trauma to the already fragile skin. The patient should contact the physician if any signs or symptoms of infection occur.

Referral to a lymphedema clinic or wound clinic well versed in lymphedema management is an excellent resource for the patient (Bryant, 2000.)

SUMMARY

The management of wounds can be complicated by many factors, both internally and externally. Generalized edema and lymphedema are considerable factors that can have detrimental effects not only on wound healing but also on maintenance of an anatomically functional limb. Generalized edema may be acute, as with trauma or surgery, or it may be chronic, as with congestive heart failure. Generalized edema can usually be managed with elevation, ice, anti-inflammatory medications, diuretics, and compression therapy. Lymphedema, on the other hand, is a result of a dysfunctional lymphatic system and can become quite chronic, leading to prolonged wound healing, poor cosmetic effect, and a dysfunctional limb. Diuretics, anti-inflammatory medications, and even elevation (in the later stages) are not as effective in treating with lymphedema. The mainstay of therapy for lymphedema is comprehensive decongestive therapy, including manual lymph drainage, compression bandaging, elevation, exercises, and patient education. The clinician needs to discuss with the patient that lymphedema is a chronic disorder that currently has no known cure. Long-term maintenance of the condition requires a continued focus on the general principles of lymphedema management and a lifetime commitment to these principles.

CHAPTER 9
Questions 73-76

73. The edema associated with lymphedema is formed by

    a. high-protein fluid remaining in the interstitial spaces.

    b. vascular insufficiency.

    c. improper diet.

    d. an abundance of lymph nodes.

74. Generalized edema is managed by

    a. use of pain medication on a routine basis.

    b. elevation of the extremity.

    c. therapeutic massage of the extremity.

    d. application of heat to the area three times a day.

75. Stage II lymphedema is characterized by

    a. fibrosis of the skin.

    b. pitting of the tissues that underlie the epidermis.

    c. edema that comes and goes without any particular treatment.

    d. chronic skin changes that often have an orange-peel appearance.

76. Lymphedema has

    a. three classifications and two stages.

    b. three classifications and three stages.

    c. two classifications and two stages.

    d. two classifications and three stages.

CHAPTER 10

WOUND MANAGEMENT

CHAPTER OBJECTIVES

Upon completion of the chapter, the reader will be able to identify factors involved in effective wound management, including wound cleansing, infection treatment, debridement, and topical wound care. The reader will also be able to discuss principles used to minimize complications and make knowledge-based decisions regarding topical product selection to achieve desired outcomes.

LEARNING OBJECTIVES

After completion of the chapter, the reader will be able to

1. differentiate between colonization of wounds and infection of wounds.

2. list ways to optimize the microenvironment of a wound.

3. discuss the four methods of debridement and their effects on wound management.

4. state the principles of selecting products to achieve a moist wound environment.

INTRODUCTION

As previously explained, wound healing is a complex cascade of events. To effectively manage a wound and achieve healing, attention to the wound's microenvironment is imperative.

Previous chapters have discussed factors that contribute to wound formation and factors that impair healing. For the most part, acute surgical wounds heal uneventfully. Chronic wounds, on the other hand, are affected by multiple factors and, due to the chronicity of these wounds, the clinician needs to understand the management of the affecting factors. Well-known impediments to wound repair are infection, pooled exudate, and necrotic tissue. To create an optimally healthy environment, topical therapy should promote a moist wound environment, challenge when coupled with the goal of preventing injury to the surrounding skin. This chapter concentrates on the management of chronic wounds. Although the local environment is the focus of discussion here, the clinician must understand that nutrition, blood flow, pressure, shearing, friction, moisture control, management of disease processes, and patient education continue to play a role in the management of wounds.

WOUND MANAGEMENT: AN HISTORICAL PERSPECTIVE

In the past, topical management of wounds has been quite varied and depended on trial and error rather than scientific evidence. Some of the past treatments for wounds include clay, honey, pine tar, feathers, waxes, oils, and moss. Even in the last 15–20 years such topical products as sugar, antacids, and bismuth have been used. As information and technology advanced, the basic foundation of topical treatment changed. Since 1962, and especially in the last 10–15 years, the focus of topical treatment and research has been based on the moist wound healing theory, which facilitates epithelial migration, enhances granulation tissue formation, and facilitates autolytic debridement of necrotic tissue (Van Rijswijk, 1996). As scientific research continues, it redirects chronic wound management to evidenced-based practice.

The moist wound healing theory caused an explosion in wound care treatment modalities and products. It is extremely difficult to adequately evaluate all of the products on their ability to assist with wound repair as well as maintain cost efficiency. No matter what the product, several principles of wound management derived from scientific studies can help to achieve positive wound outcomes. Manufacturers try to fit their products into one or more of these principles

- Treat infection

- Debride necrotic tissue

- Prevent premature wound closure

- Absorb excess exudate

- Maintain moist environment

- Provide insulation

- Protect from reinjury and contamination.

INFECTION

Colonization and contamination are common phenomena in chronic wounds. For the purposes of this discussion, these two terms will be used synonymously. Colonization is defined as the presence of microbes without infection. Microbes are everywhere; they colonize the body and the environment. The skin and body orifices are heavily colonized with microbes, with fewer numbers found deep within the body. Infection occurs when the tissue is invaded by microbes and destruction of the cells occurs (Krasner & Kane, 2001). Health care providers must understand the difference between colonization and infection to determine the plan of care for a patient.

Colonized wounds have a high bacterial count on the wound surface, commonly referred to as a bacterial load or bioburden. The goal in treatment of these wounds is to decrease the amount of bacteria so that the host can better manage the load, therefore preventing infection. One way to accomplish this is by aggressive irrigation, which removes and dilutes the bacteria on the wound surface. Cleansing the wound by irrigation at a dressing change or having the patient shower are acceptable methods of removing the surface bacteria.

Infection results from the inability of the host to manage the bacterial load of the wound (see Figure 10-1). White blood cells are unable to manage the number of microbes and the progression to infection begins. However, a lower count of microbes can also cause infection in the presence of impaired

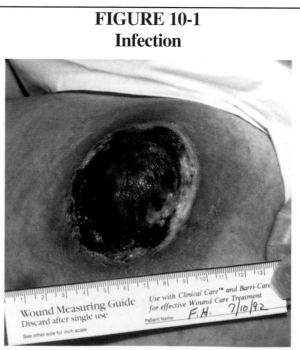

FIGURE 10-1
Infection

Trochanter wound with local infection leading to systemic infection. Note the erythema around the wound. Physical examination revealed warmth, induration, odor, and purulent drainage.

blood flow or a compromised host. This impairment of blood flow can be either from arterial insufficiency or from pressure.

How does the clinician determine if a wound is colonized or infected? Clinical signs found in the assessment and wound trends can assist the clinician in determining if infection is present. Local infection is determined by the four classic signs rubor (redness), calor (heat), dolor (pain), and tumor (swelling). As infection advances into surrounding tissue, cellulitis occurs. A wound that shows signs of deterioration (such as an increase in pain or changes in the amount, odor, or color of exudate) should alert the clinician to possible infection.

An understanding of wound products is also essential when differentiating infection from colonization. Topical therapy that enhances autolysis of nonviable tissue increases the amount of exudate and mimics the appearance of pus. If the topical dressing is occlusive, it will change the odor of the wound due to the anaerobic environment. Without this basic knowledge, mistakes are easily made and chronic wounds are overtreated.

If infection is suspected, a wound culture is indicated. The type of culture performed determines the accuracy of the results. The literature supports several clinically acceptable methods of obtaining samples for culture, including

• surface swab

• needle aspiration

• curettage of the ulcer base

• tissue biopsy.

The surface swab, or swab culture, is the most readily available method. This method requires the lowest level of skill and is accessible to acute care, long term care, clinics, and home health. The most accurate in identifying the pathogen responsible for the infection is the tissue biopsy; since this is classified as a biopsy, it limits the procedure to advanced level clinicians and physicians. Wound swab cul-

tures may detect colonizing bacteria rather than pathogens but, with proper technique, can closely approximate tissue biopsy. There are two techniques generally accepted for obtaining a swab culture; both require a thorough cleansing of the wound bed with sterile normal saline solution or water. The culture should be obtained either by pressing gently on the surrounding skin to expel deep exudate or by rotating a sterile swab in a 1-cm area of the wound for 5 seconds, using slight pressure to cause minimal bleeding. The clinician should avoid necrotic tissue because it is known to be polymicrobial.

Another technique, needle aspiration, tends to be more accurate as compared to deep tissue biopsy but can underestimate the actual number of organisms (Maklebust & Sieggreen, 2001). The results obtained by curettage of the ulcer base show the best correlation with deep tissue biopsy. However, many clinicians do not have the luxury of these choices for determining infection and for identifying the organism. If the only method available is swab culture, a few principles should be followed to minimize the risk of contamination. The clinician should first cleanse the wound well with saline, dry it, and then choose one of the two methods above to obtain the specimen.

When interpreting culture results, the clinician is looking for 1) the type of microbe and 2) the amount of the microbe. The amount, or colony count, that causes an infection varies depending on the host. The general guideline, based on several studies, is that a colony count greater than 100,000 organisms/gm of tissue (10^5) impairs wound healing (AHCPR, 1994). At this level, the body is no longer able to manage the load of microbes and wound healing is impaired. Depending on the host's condition, a lesser count could inhibit wound healing or cause infection. Remember, the step before infection is a balancing act. What amount of bacteria can the host, or patient, manage in the wound environment before bacteria overload the host's ability to control the invasion of tissues? It should be noted that this guideline does not hold true for B-hemolytic streptococcus, which can impair or prevent healing with colony counts of less than 10^5 (Bryant, 2000). There are also studies reporting that approximately 25% of nonhealing pressure ulcers have underlying osteomyelitis (AHCPR, 1994). Suspicion of osteomyelitis should lead to further investigation. Obtaining a bone biopsy is recommended to identify the organism and effectively treat osteomyelitis.

The prudent use of antibiotics is necessary to avoid drug-resistant organisms. The prevalence of the resistant pathogens methicillin-resistant *Staphylococcus aureus* (MRSA) and vancomycin-resistant *Enterococcus* (VRE) is increasing. Prevention and control of the spread of these organisms requires the coordinated efforts of all health care workers. Education on controlling the spread of these pathogens should be given to all health care workers. Those caring for wounds can assist by using standard precautions and by employing aseptic technique in wound care. Supporting the host's resistance against pathogens can also assist in infection control. The use of comprehensive skills to differentiate contamination from infection in a wound and the use of proper culturing technique to prevent erroneous use of antibiotics help to decrease the potential of other microorganisms developing antibiotic resistance.

WOUND CLEANSING

Optimal wound healing cannot proceed until surface contaminants, slough, necrotic debris, foreign bodies, purulent exudate, and bacteria are removed. Selection of the wound cleansing solution should be based on the effects of that solution on wound healing. Safety and efficacy of wound cleansers has not yet been critically scrutinized by the U.S. Food and Drug Administration (FDA). Antiseptic solutions were the standard for many years but are now known to have detrimental effects on cells and tissues and, at times, even on intact skin. The use of antiseptics in reducing up to 95% of bacteria on skin before procedures has been well documented (Sussman & Bates-Jensen, 2004). There is not, however, a considerable amount of definitive research on the effects in wounds. The issue with their use is cell toxicity as well as interference with collagen deposition. Acetic acid, povidone-iodine, sodium hypochlorite, and hydrogen peroxide are all cytotoxic to fibroblasts and should be avoided. The most readily available, cost-effective, and tissue friendly cleansing solution is isotonic saline (0.9% sodium chloride). It can be used safely for treatments ranging from gentle cleansing on a clean granulating wound to irrigating with enough force to cleanse contaminated wounds. When wounds are heavily contaminated, the clinician can use larger amounts of solution to flush and dilute the contaminates. Although the literature supports the fact that antiseptics are cytotoxic, there is still controversy in the wound care community. Some clinicians support that antiseptics should never be used and others cannot be convinced to end their use after so many years. The authors of this book have occasionally used antiseptics in the presence of infection or a highly contaminated, foul-smelling wound when the wound bed had a non-viable wound base (therefore, not damaging any fibroblasts). The use of antiseptics was limited to 3 days, which the authors believe can assist in decreasing bacterial load and controlling exudate and odor in the wound until antibiotic levels can attain therapeutic levels.

Acetic acid is used against *Pseudomonas* species (as well as other aerobic gram-negative rods) because these organisms show a marked sensitivity to this solution. It is particularly effective because these organisms do not penetrate tissue deeply and can be cleared with topical therapy. Once again, treatment should be limited but can be useful for *Pseudomonas,* which is apt to develop antimicrobial resistance. Brief vinegar soaks or compresses for 15 minutes per day may be preferable to antibiotic therapy if significant invasion has not taken place (Krasner & Kane, 2001). Hypochlorites (Dakin's solution, for example), are chemically unstable and deactivated by organic material and blood in the wound. They may have a role in the treatment of an ischemic limb, where controlling odor and the spread of infection are the goals of treatment. Povodine-iodine solution is bactericidal and sporicidal, but local irritation and sensitivity can occur and, with large wounds, the absorption rate can interfere with thyroid function tests. In general, the use of topical antiseptics in chronic wounds has limited benefit and may be injurious to tissues. Most investigators call for further research in this area to assist in directing their use in chronic wound care. Because acute wounds differ from chronic wounds, acute wounds can benefit from the use of antiseptics to reduce the level of bacteria. But once again, there is controversy in the literature. An exception for chronic wound use is in the immunocompromised patient or when poor arterial circulation is present. The dressing that has shown to be the exception with chronic wounds is cadexomer iodine. Although the product is an iodine, it is different than povodine-iodine, because it has 0.9% iodine trapped within a three-dimensional starch lattice. As exudate is absorbed into this dressing a small amount of the iodine is released. Slow release of this antimicrobial agent allows for the maintenance of low iodine levels, thereby reducing bacteria levels over time. Numerous studies support its use in the treatment of chronic wounds.

Wound assessment also helps in the decision-making process; if the wound base is necrotic, an antiseptic solution cannot harm the tissue. If a granulation base is present, yet you suspect a bacterial burden, you must consider ways to decrease the bacteria count. As mentioned before, cleansing with volume, regardless of solution, may be all that is needed. When using any antiseptic, the clinician must understand the risks and benefits of ordering a particular treatment.

The other option available for wound cleansing is a surfactant wound cleanser. This may be a better option when using light scrubbing in the cleansing process. The surfactant decreases trauma to the wound tissue. Saline has a minimal ability to reduce frictional forces on the wound tissue during scrubbing. The surfactants reduce that coefficient of friction (Krasner & Kane, 2001). In making decisions regarding the use of cleansers and antiseptics, the clinician should be aware of the detrimental effects on cells and any other contraindications specific to their use.

The mechanical force of the liquid used for wound cleansing is important to the outcomes of wound management. The amount of force to use on the wound tissue during irrigation depends on the method selected. The *AHCPR Clinical Practice Guidelines: Treatment of Pressure Ulcers* states that 4–15 psi irrigation pressures are safe and effective. Irrigation pressures of commonly used methods are as follows: bulb syringe at 2 psi; piston syringe with catheter tip at 4.2 psi; 35-ml syringe with 19-gauge needle or angiocath at 8 psi; 12-ml syringe with 22-gauge needle at 13 psi; and water-pik on lowest setting at 6.0 psi. One human study that compared the bulb syringe (2 psi) irrigation of acute wounds to the 12-ml syringe with a 22-gauge needle (13 psi) showed less wound inflammation and wound infection for wounds cleansed with syringe and needle irrigation. The water-pik at the middle setting (#3) is 42 psi and the highest setting (#5) is > 50 psi.

Because of the high pressures, these methods should not be used in general wound care. The use of high pressure has been documented to disperse fluid into adjacent tissue or along tissue plains (Krasner & Kane, 2001). The irrigation of wounds has been made more convenient by the introduction of battery-powered self-contained irrigation systems. Experimental studies comparing pulsatile or continuous flow have not documented the superiority of either method. The important component seems to be the pressure of the stream. The clinician needs to check with the manufacturer of any product or device that claims to deliver pressurized irrigation about the impact the system delivers to the wound bed. The goal is to deliver between 4–15 psi until further studies direct us toward understanding the best wound irrigation to remove debris while sparing healthy wound tissue.

The *AHCPR Clinical Practice Guidelines* also recommend whirlpool for cleansing pressure ulcers that contain thick exudate, slough, or necrotic tis-sue. Several studies have also demonstrated effective wound cleansing of venous stasis ulcers with whirlpool followed by 30 seconds of rinsing at the maximum force tolerated. However, once the wound has been cleansed of foreign debris, the benefits of the whirlpool are outweighed by the trauma to the newly exposed healing tissue (Krasner, 2001). Therefore, discontinue treatment when the ulcer is clean and do not expose clean granulating wounds to whirlpool therapy.

TABLE 10-1
TYPES OF DEBRIDEMENT

Type	Characteristics	Advantages	Disadvantages
Sharp	• Use of a scalpel, scissors, or other sharp instrument to remove devitalized tissue • To remove areas of thick, adherent eschar and devitalized tissue	• Quickest form of debridement • Removes necrotic tissue quickly in presence of infection • Selective,** if not down to bleeding base	• Requires skilled clinician • May require trip to OR • Nonselective* • May be painful
Mechanical	• Hydrotherapy (whirlpool or pulse lavage) & irrigation: soften and/or remove devitalized tissue and debris through mechanical force • 4-15 psi irrigation pressures are considered safe and effective (without trauma to viable tissue)	• Assists in control of bacterial load • Can achieve an 8 psi with a 35ml syringe and 19-gauge angiocath irrigation	• Nonselective* • Can be painful • Cost of treatment • Psi <4 is ineffective • Psi >15 can be harmful to granulating tissue, may drive bacteria into tissue
	• Wet-to-dry dressings are removed dry to remove devitalized tissue • Partly defeats function if dressing is moistened before removal • Discontinue when wound is clean	• Readily available • Easy dressing changes	• Nonselective* • Frequent dressing changes (q4-6 hrs) not cost-efficient for home health agencies • Can be painful
Enzymatic (Chemical)	• Application of topical enzyme (proteolytic, fibrinolytic, collangenase) that digests necrotic tissue • Not as effective with dry eschar, enzyme will not penetrate dry surface	• Selective** • Utilized when unable to tolerate sharp or mechanical • Applied once a day • Minimal pain • No skill involved	• Some may cause stinging • Slower than sharp or mechanical • Can increase wound drainage as liquefaction occurs • Requires prescription
Autolytic	• Use of a moist wound environment to allow devitalized tissue to self-digest from enzymes normally present in wound fluids • When unable to tolerate other forms of debridement or for patients who are not likely to become infected with a slower debridement	• Selective,** most sparing to viable tissue • No pain • Available to all patients	• May take longer than other debridement forms • Can increase wound drainage as liquefaction occurs • Not effective for large amounts of necrotic tissue

* Nonselective — removes tissue regardless of viability
** Selective — removes only necrotic tissue

DEBRIDEMENT

Necrotic tissue, a source for bacterial overgrowth, must be removed to optimize wound healing and prevent the occurrence of infection. Areas of necrotic tissue can mask underlying fluid or abscesses. Debridement is the removal of nonviable tissue (eschar, slough or fibrin) or nonviable structures (bone or tendon). Debridement of nonviable tissue is an important factor in the management of contaminated wounds. Debridement provides a vascular and viable wound environment to set the stage for granulation and wound contraction to occur. The type of debridement chosen depends on several factors: the speed at which removal is needed, the type of tissue involved, the amount of tissue, and the methods available to the clinician. Methods of debridement are: sharp, mechanical, chemical, and autolytic (see Table 10-1).

Sharp

Sharp debridement is the removal of necrotic or devitalized tissue using a sharp, sterile instrument, such as a scissors, scalpel, or laser. Sharp debridement, although the fastest method of debridement, is not always readily available in all settings. Sharp debridement can be performed at the bedside or in the operating room. When performed in the operating room, it is referred to as surgical debridement. These terms are often used interchangeably because at times the same instruments are used at the bedside. The presence of infection necessitates immediate removal of necrotic tissue and sharp debridement is indicated. In the presence of large amounts of necrotic tissue, the length of time required to accomplish the goal of removal by more conservative means of debridement is unrealistic, sharp debridement should be the method of choice (see Figures 10-2 and 10-3). Depending on the setting, the status of the wound, and the patient's status, a physician or surgeon, physical therapist, or certified wound nurse can perform sharp debridement. Clinicians other than physicians should check with their respective state licensing boards to determine their scope of practice and any requirements or restrictions that may pertain to debridement. Clinicians should consider performing debridement under a specified protocol.

FIGURE 10-2
Abdominal Wound: Anterior View

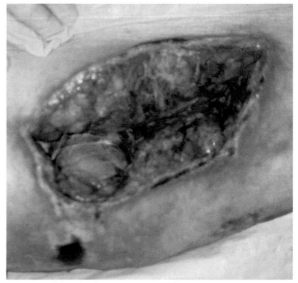

Status post wound infection, dehiscence, and debridement. A polysaccharide starch absorption dressing was used, which decreased dressing frequency and pain, and promoted autolysis.

FIGURE 10-3
Abdominal Wound: Inferior View

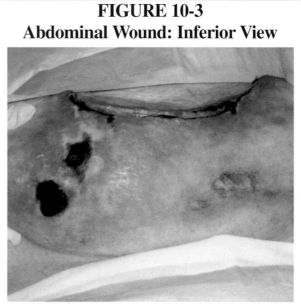

Inferior side of the wound in Figure 10-2 after eschar was debrided; communication to the main wound was then evident.

Mechanical

Mechanical debridement can be accomplished in many ways; the most common is the wet-to-dry dressing. A wet-to-dry dressing is designed to adhere to necrotic tissue as it dries. The tissue imbeds itself into the loosely woven gauze; upon removal of the dressing, the necrotic tissue is removed from the wound bed. It is a nonselective method of debridement, meaning that it can not differentiate between tissue types, viable or nonviable. Potential harm to any granulation tissue in the wound base is possible each time the dressing is removed. Pain can also be a significant issue. Although necrotic tissue has no responding pain receptors, the pulling on underlying tissue can cause significant pain to the patient. To minimize pain, clinicians commonly dampen the dressing prior to removal which, to varying degrees, diminishes the effect of debridement. Whirlpool, pulse lavage, scrubbing of the wound bed, and irrigation are also methods to mechanically remove necrotic tissue in a wound. Once again, remember the recommended psi for mechanical removal of necrotic tissue is 4–15. Several methods are available, as discussed in this chapter.

Chemical

Chemical debridement with enzymatic agents is a selective method of debridement (see Figure 10-4). Various types of enzymes target specific necrotic tissues, such as protein, fibrin, and collagen. Necrotic fibrins and proteins are located in the wound bed more superficially than devitalized collagen. The enzymatic agents available at the time of this writing are applied daily and can be covered with dry gauze, a nonadherent dressing, or with some wound products. The goal in selecting a secondary dressing is to keep the wound bed moist and prevent the enzyme from drying out, which inactivates the chemical. When treating dry, thick eschar the enzyme is not as effective due to the difficulty of getting the enzyme through the thick surface and to the moist area

below. Some clinicians cross-hatch the eschar to promote penetration through the thick, hard surface. This is still an extremely slow and expensive method for debriding dry eschar covered wounds. An alternative method to debridement should be considered at this point. Also, be sure to read the package insert because some cleansers and dressings with metal components, such as sulfadiazine, can inactivate the enzyme. Chemical debridement, as with other forms of extrinsic debridement, needs to be discontinued when the wound bed is free from necrotic tissue.

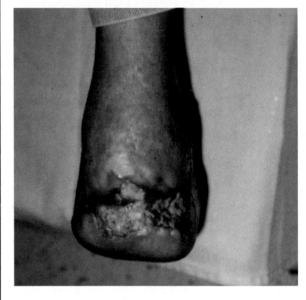

FIGURE 10-4
Transmetatarsal Amputation

Transmetatarsal amputation with necrotic suture line. Poor response to sharp debridement secondary to arterial insufficiency. Responded well to slow enzymatic debridement.

Autolytic

Autolysis, an intrinsic debridement, is the purest form of selective debridement — the use of the body's own enzymes to digest devitalized tissue. The wound fluid, which is full of macrophages and neutrophils, digests and liquefies necrotic tissue. Although it is the most selective method and has the least incidence of pain, it is a slower form of debridement.

Autolytic debridement is accomplished by providing a moist environment over the wound bed, which in itself facilitates the autolytic process (see Figures 10-5 & 10-6). It is often used as an adjunct to other methods of debridement or when low levels or adherent slough is present. This method is appropriate for patients who are unable to tolerate other methods of debridement or when there is not a high risk of infection if more rapid methods are not utilized.

The choice of debridement depends on a multitude of factors. Each form has its own unique characteristics, and often more than one form is used on a wound as the dynamics of the wound change. The decision is based on the type of wound, the accessibility of various methods, the condition of the patient, the patient setting, the caregiver's ability, and the financial burden. The primary goal is ridding the wound of necrotic tissue to maximize wound healing.

FIGURE 10-5
Stage III Pressure Ulcer

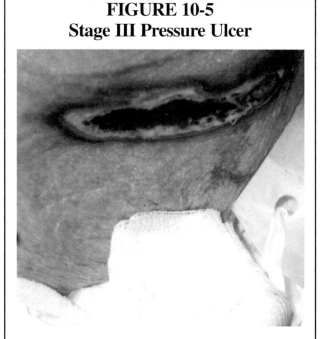

Stage III pressure ulcer in lateral lumbar/buttock region secondary to a halo brace. Wound bed: 75% granulation tissue and 25% slough. Status after sharp debridement, pressure relief and moist wound healing. Hydrogel dressings to continue with autolytic debridement.

FIGURE 10-6
Stage III Pressure Ulcer Follow-up

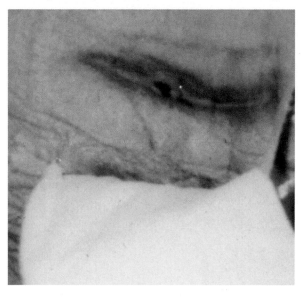

Follow-up of Stage III pressure ulcer in Figure 10-5 as treatment continued.

MOIST WOUND HEALING

Moist wound healing is the area of wound care that receives the most attention. The primary goal of local wound management is to keep the wound bed moist and the surrounding skin dry. The microenvironment of the wound bed needs to be optimized to promote the wound healing cascade (see Figure 10-7). In chronic wounds, this can become sluggish. Although a great deal of precedence is given to the choice of wound care product, it is a small fraction of the total wound management picture. The clinician may look at the enormous selection of wound care products available and become overwhelmed, making product selection somewhat difficult.

Wound care products can generally be separated into generic categories based on the amount of exudate control. Does the product add moisture to the wound or absorb exudate? There is no wound dressing available that will treat all wounds. Before studying these generic categories, the clinician must realize it is impossible to include all variations of

FIGURE 10-7
Stage III Pressure Ulcer from Prosthesis

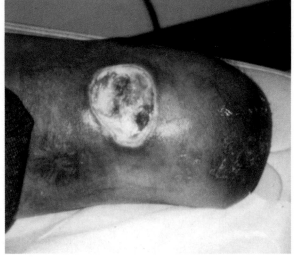

Stage III pressure ulcer from a prosthetic device. Patient had been fitted for the prosthesis 8 years earlier and never had the device re-evaluated. Treated with sharp debridement and Hydrogel with good results.

products. There is a continual flood of new products into the market each year, including those that combine various product features in different formulations. These products, referred to as "combination products," are presented to the market each day and change as the industry tries to meet the growing needs of clinicians. This plethora of products is both exciting and overwhelming, giving clinicians more choices to accomplish the goals of an ideal wound environment. The recommendation is for the clinician to learn the generic categories. Then, as the clinician becomes more comfortable with using these categories, the unique variations of individual products will find a place in the clinician's arsenal of options.

No wound with significant tissue loss is treated with the same product throughout the entire healing process. So, what decision-making process does the clinician proceed with to choose the appropriate dressing product for a particular wound? First in the decision-making process is consideration of the

assessment, using it to dictate your choice of dressing. Ask these questions: What does the wound look like? What type of tissue is present? Are signs of infection present? What type and amount of exudate is on the previous dressing? The wound assessment should dictate the goal for the subsequent dressing. Is there necrotic tissue that needs to be removed? Does granulation tissue line the wound bed and need a gentle, friendly environment to continue proliferation? A knowledge of the characteristics of the dressing, the type of wound bed present, and the expectation of outcomes can greatly assist the clinician. The mixing and matching of the wound to the dressing is important to understand. For instance, when the dressing is expected to enhance autolysis, the clinician should anticipate an increase of drainage. Does it require a more absorptive secondary dressing? Should the dressing be changed twice a day initially to accommodate for the increased drainage? Does the surrounding skin need protection? Foresight by the clinician can alleviate potential problems for both the patient and staff. In addition, the clinician must be aware that liquefaction of nonviable tissue with autolytic debridement mimics the appearance of pus. Also, if an occlusive dressing is used, the clinician should know that an odor will be present when it is removed, because it is in an anaerobic environment. The clinician should warn the family and patient as well as other staff. When the first hydrocolloids were introduced, they were occlusive dressings (today most are semiocclusive). Many physicians were alarmed when removing dressings in their offices, and would discontinue the dressing because they suspected infection. Once again, knowledge is imperative not only for the clinician selecting the dressing but for all people involved in wound care. Communication is key; some needs to be documented and other information can be passed verbally. Informing the patient or caregiver what is happening also allows them to pass on the information to new clinicians involved in their care.

Generally, when there is dead space in a wound, it needs to be obliterated. There may be instances when filling dead space is not justified; however, for this discussion, assume that the goal is to eliminate dead space. Dead space promotes pooling of exudate, which can increase the bacterial load and early closing at the surface. Packing needs to obliterate the dead space without creating excessive pressure within the wound. Tight packing may be needed initially after sharp debridement to control the bleeding. Tight packing can cause pressure on the wound bed and impede blood flow to the tissue. The goal of packing is to wick exudate out of the wound to the secondary dressing. This eliminates pooling and the risk of increasing bacterial loads. A challenge presents when there is a tract with a small skin opening. In this case, it is difficult to insert packing material and also to ensure that it is completely removed.

Second in the decision-making process is the dressing itself. When removing a dressing from a wound the clinician should take the time to observe. Each dressing tells a story that helps the clinician make an informed decision on treatment choices. Was the dressing completely saturated? If so, was the surrounding skin exposed to exudate for a period of time? Did the dressing create an excessively moist environment that overhydrated the skin and caused damage? Or was the dressing dry and adhering to the wound bed? All of these factors tell the clinician how the wound is responding to the management and what needs to be accomplished. The choice of dressing should be an informed decision.

Many factors are considered when choosing the appropriate dressing. Is there a willing and able caregiver? The caregiver may be willing to place a superficial dressing on after a shower, but can he or she assist when the wound care involves irrigation of a tunnel or a wound with depth? Once again, communication with the caregiver is important, not only with instructing how to change the dressing but also on what to expect upon dressing removal. Consider the patient care setting: is the patient at home or in a

health care setting with trained staff performing care? Is the environment clean? The dressing choice may protect the wound from the environment. Many times a dressing that has a semipermeable membrane may be chosen for a wound in the perineal region when a patient is not continent. It may also be the dressing of choice when the house is unclean and the patient may be exposed to a large number of contaminants. If infection is present, dressing changes are generally more frequent. Long-wear dressings should not be used when twice a day dressing changes are required. The location of the ulcer also plays a role. How is an adhesive dressing to adhere to it? Will the dressing stay on in this area? How will this dressing perform under pressure, for example, the pressure under a compression wrap? Is the dressing appropriate for a paraplegic sitting in a wheelchair? Is the choice of dressing on a foot wound going to add pressure when the patient puts on his shoe? The location and the patient's activity influence the clinician's choice of dressing. The availability of dressings from the contracted supplier may also dictate what is available or how quickly clinicians can special order a product. In some settings, the payment source also changes the availability of products. The accumulation of all this information is utilized in the decision-making process, matching the dressing to the wound to achieve the desired outcome. The evaluation of dressing effectiveness is a key factor in wound care. Has the wound responded the way you wanted? Is the dressing performance adequate? Remember, wound monitoring at regular intervals assists the clinician in assessing the progress of the wound. Wounds are dynamic and, therefore, topical dressing selection changes as the needs of the wound change.

PERIWOUND INJURIES

Sometimes, when a wound is treated, the skin surrounding that wound (the periwound skin) is injured. Because periwound skin is a part of the wound assessment, it plays a role in the decision of a wound dressing. Skin tears, erosions, and denuded skin are the most common periwound injuries. Treatment of these injuries should adhere to the same principles as the primary dressing goal: to maintain a moist wound environment, protect the wound and surrounding skin, and control exudate.

Skin tears occur when the dermoepidermal junction is separated. This junction is weakened with aging, making elderly patients much more susceptible to this type of injury. Skin tears are fairly common on the arms of elderly patients (see Figure 10-8). Another population vulnerable to this injury are steroid-dependent patients. Skin tear is a catch-all term for several skin injuries, although each has a varying etiology. Their treatments are similar because each lead to a similar injury: epidermal loss. Skin tears, skin stripping, and tension blisters (commonly called tape blisters) all fall into this category.

FIGURE 10-8
Skin Tear

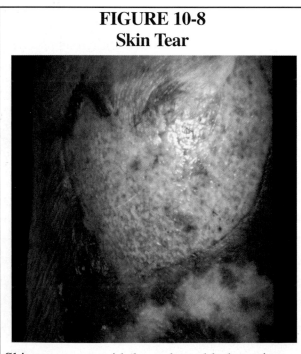

Skin tear on steroid-dependent elderly patient.

Once a tear occurs, treatment is determined based on the location of the tear. Depending on the drainage, there are several treatment options for skin tears on the arms. A fine- or wide-mesh impregnated gauze can be used. The wide mesh allows passage of fluid more readily. The impregnated gauze can be covered with roll gauze and changed every day to every other day, depending on the amount of drainage. Another option for treatment is the use of an ointment covered by a nonadherent secondary dressing. These are both nonadherant options. There are many more nonadherant dressings available, for example, hydrogel sheets and nonadhesive foams. Hydrogel sheets absorb little; foams, however, absorb much more fluid but do so slowly and may not manage the fluid of a skin tear on an edematous arm adequately. The second option is adhesive dressings. For example, some clinicians choose polyurethane films. Caution needs to be taken with these dressings, though, because their adhesive property can further damage the skin. If a polyurethane film is utilized, there should be minimal drainage, and the clinician should anticipate that the dressing can stay on for a long period of time. As long as healing continues, this type of dressing should be left in place. Wound fluid eventually evaporates because of the semipermeable property of these dressings allows the passage of vapor. As time passes, the normal sloughing of epidermal cells occurs and the dressing can easily be removed without reinjury or extension of the skin tear. The difficulty with polyurethane films is keeping the dressing in place; both health care workers and family members have a hard time leaving the dressing untouched.

Another important consideration in choosing a dressing is the nature of the wound, periwounds are usually acute injuries, not chronic nonhealing wounds. Dressing choices differ in an acute care setting versus a home care or outpatient setting. Is it feasible to change the dressing everyday at home like it is in the ICU setting? Probably not. The use of advanced dressings is often clinically appropriate but may not be economically prudent; all factors need to be considered.

Skin stripping is a term used when the epidermal layer is pulled off by adhesive dressings or tape. Frequent tape removal is the most common cause, with an increased risk in the presence of fragile skin. Each time tape is removed, it removes the top layer of sloughing epidermal cells. One can visualize this when transparent tape, used for taping papers, is removed from the skin. The sloughing of cells is a normal process; however, repeated adhesive applications, the supply of sloughing cells is exhausted and stripping of the healthy protective layer of skin begins to occur. An adhesive primary dressing can also cause skin stripping from the strength of the adhesive, known as the aggressiveness of the adhesive. Most adhesive dressings are designed for extended wear, and the adhesive aggressiveness decreases with time. Therefore, it is less likely to create a skin injury if removed on day 3 or 4 versus day 1. This is another important reason to know your dressing expectation. Ask yourself: how much will the dressing absorb and what do I expect from this wound? Will this adhesive dressing last a few days? What is the condition of the periwound skin? A clinician can have two similar wounds to care for but choose two different wound products based on the condition of the periwound skin.

Tension blisters, commonly referred to as tape blisters, can result in loss of the epidermal layer. These are most commonly seen under tape that secures a dressing to an initial postoperative abdominal wound or a postoperative pressure dressing. These skin tears can result within the initial 24–48 hours after surgery. As postoperative edema causes tension on the dermoepidermal junction, a blister forms and creates a weakened state. Upon removal of the tape and dressing, the epidermis is torn off, leaving the resultant injury, a skin tear. Early removal of the surgical dressing and retaping without tension can help decrease the chances of injury. If the surgeon does not want the dressing removed, the clinician may be permitted to loosen and trim the tape to reduce tension. If the original surgical dressing is removed and skin tears are found in the tape area of the dressing, the area needs to be protected from the trauma of tape removal. A hydrocolloid can

be placed over the area to create a base for taping. Montgomery straps can also be used over the hydrocolloid to increase the weartime of the hydrocolloid and prevent pulling on the adhesion. This same treatment should be instituted to prevent injury.

The damage to skin from adhesive products can be avoided by diligent assessment. Can a different dressing type be used to decrease the frequency of dressing change? Is the skin showing signs of preinjury such as erythema, or does the patient complain of discomfort? The use of a skin sealant can help decrease the incidence of skin injury, especially skin stripping. These products provide a clear, protective layer on the skin. When tape is removed, it removes this layer of sealant rather than stripping the epidermal layer. It is an excellent preventive measure but should be used cautiously with broken skin because it may contain alcohol as a base. There are products available with a silicone base that allow use on broken or irritated skin without discomfort. The use of nonadhesive secondary dressings can avoid taping on the skin. A dressing can be anchored down with gauze roll or by placing adhesive products beyond the area at risk. If an adhesive product is needed, an adhesive remover may be helpful in reducing the incidence of skin tearing during removal. The best treatment for any type of skin tear, however, is early prevention. Prevention is a proactive approach resulting from assessment, evaluation, and knowledge of the potential injuries and the choices for interventions available to the clinician.

The periwound skin can also be damaged by excessive moisture. Skin which is normally dry, is the body's first line of defense. When it is exposed to excessive moisture, overhydration of the epidermis occurs, leading to softening and disintegration. The most familiar example is dish-pan hands from submersion in water. Maceration can result from soaking in water, perspiration, incontinence, wound exudate, or dressing moisture. The periwound maceration discussed here is related to wound exudate or moist dressings (see Figure 10-9).

FIGURE 10-9
Sacral Coccyx

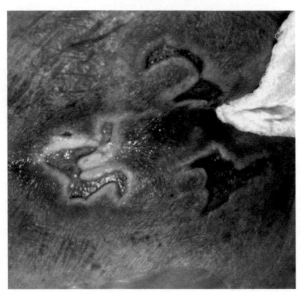

Multiple shear wounds with macerated wound edges. A change of treatment is indicated, such as more absorptive dressing or a barrier to protect the wound edges from moisture. Note the edge of the hydrocolloids seen at the bottom of the photo, these were used on each buttock to prevent tape injury to the skin.

Maceration related to wounds is managed in two ways: 1) management of the moisture and 2) protection of the skin. To manage moisture, the clinician can change the type of dressing or increase the frequency of dressing change. Is the dressing used too wet, adding excessive moisture to the area? A wet-to-dry dressing or a moist saline dressing applied to the wound can rest on the periwound skin and bathe it in moisture until the next dressing change. A hydrogel dressing, containing mostly water, adds moisture to the area. When a wound is superficial or small, the dressing can affect the periwound skin as well as the wound bed. When maceration occurs with an adhesive dressing such as a hydrocolloid, resolution may be accomplished by selecting a foam product. Protecting the skin is the next step. Simply adding the use of a skin moisture barrier on the periwound skin can protect it from maceration. Creams or ointments are classified as moisture barriers when their active ingredient is petrolatum, zinc oxide, or dimethicone. Cover the periwound skin with a barrier at each dressing change. To adequately manage maceration, a more absorptive dressing may be required in addition to the use of a skin barrier.

Excessive moisture may progress beyond maceration to further erode or denude the skin. At this point, a break in the skin and diffuse erythema may be visible. Irritant or perineal dermatitis, inflammatory responses of the skin to an offending substance (such as liquid stool, urine, G-tube drainage, or wound exudate), results in erythema, erosions, denuded tissue, and pain. Treatment for this condition is basically the same. The type of barrier chosen may vary depending on the weepiness of the skin. If an adhesive dressing has been used, a non-adhesive dressing may be indicated even if it requires more frequent dressing changes. This change may be temporary, until the skin clears and can tolerate and maintain the seal of an adhesive dressing. As periwound skin becomes more permeable, the risk of developing secondary infections increases. *Candida*, a yeast, is a common opportunistic pathogen. Because this organism prefers warm, moist environments, it is easy to understand the presence of this problem when excessive moisture from wound drainage collects under a dressing. The risk of yeast is also increased when the normal flora are altered in systemic antibiotic therapy or in an immunocompromised host.

Recognizing the problem is the first step in resolution; when followed by interventions based on a knowledge of product characteristics, the goals of wound care management should be achieved.

WOUND CARE PRODUCTS BY CATEGORIES

The list of wound care products presented here is not all-inclusive, but rather, a broad sampling of what is available. Wound products are categorized according to several factors including, but not limited to, how they affect wound healing, management of the wound environment, and reimbursement guidelines (see Table 10-2). Understanding the generic categories can help the clinician choose the appropriate product for the wound characteristics. A thorough understanding of the categories is needed. It is, however, also important to evaluate each individual product, because each product in a category may be different in its composition and performance. As more complex and combination dressings become available, the clinician needs to assess each product using knowledge of the generic category to find out whether that combination is useful for a given patient. Remember that what may be true in theory may not make a difference in the overall outcome. A good analogy can be made to the use of anti-aging products. Although antiaging substances have shown to decrease wrinkles in studies, the question is, what amount does it take to accomplish that goal? In many cases, the product does not come close to the amount needed, but manufacturers can put in a small amount and claim antiaging substances are present in the product. The medical community does have more restrictions than the cosmetic industry, but one must also be aware that marketing is a lucrative business investment. Therefore, understanding products helps in the decision-making and evaluation process for wound product selection.

A more complete listing of wound products can be found in *Kestrel Wound Product Sourcebook* (Motta, 2003), an annual directory of products used for the prevention and treatment of chronic wounds.

ANTISEPTICS/TOPICAL DISINFECTANTS

Action

The value of antiseptics before procedures has been well documented; antiseptics reduce up to 95% of bacteria on the skin (Sussman & Bates-Jensen, 2004). There is not, however, a considerable amount of definitive research on the effects in wounds. The issue with their use is cell toxicity as well as interference with collagen deposition. Hypochlorites, for example, are chemically unstable and deactivated by organic material and blood in the wound. Povodine-iodine solution is bactericidal and sporicidal, but local irritation and sensitivity can occur and, with large wounds, the absorption rate can interfere with thyroid function tests. In general, the use of topical antiseptics in chronic wounds has limited benefit and may be injurious to tissues. Most investigators call for further research in this area to assist in directing their use in chronic wound care.

Acute wounds benefit from the use of antiseptics to reduce the level of bacteria. An exception for chronic wound use is in an immunocompromised patient or when poor arterial circulation is present. The dressing that has shown to be the exception with a chronic wound is the cadexomer iodine. As exudate is absorbed into this dressing, small amounts of the iodine that is trapped in the starch dressing are released. The slow release of this antimicrobial agent allows for the maintenance of low iodine levels, thereby reducing bacteria levels over time.

Indications

Antiseptics/topical disinfectants are indicated when wound bacteria levels are high and the patient is at high risk for infection. Most solutions are cytotoxic and careful consideration should be given to their use and the duration of treatment. The wound assessment helps in that decision-making process; if the wound base is necrotic, the antiseptic solution does not harm the tissue, but if a granulation base is present with a bacterial burden, you must consider

TABLE 10-2
BASIC WOUND CARE PRODUCTS

Objective	Type of Dressing	Characteristics	Type of Debridement	Precautions/Comments	Type of Wound	HCFA Usage Guidelines
Hydrate	Hydrogels Carrasyn Saf-Gel Solosite	• Formulation of waters, polymers, and other ingredients • Donates moisture to a wound or maintains moist environment • Available as amorphous gels, impregnated gauze, or sheets • Atraumatic and conform to wound bed	Autolytic	• Can dry a shallow wound; avoid by adjusting secondary dressing • May cause transient stinging to sensitive wounds • Not appropriate for high-exudate wounds • Consider as an alternative to wet-to-dry dressing	• All open wounds	Daily
	Transparent film or TAD** Tegaderm OpSite BlisterFilm CarraFilm	• Adhesive, semipermeable*, polyurethane membrane dressing • Moisture retentive by inhibiting excessive vapor loss from the wound • Provides a protective covering against shear and friction • Secondary dressing • Promotes granulation, epithelialization, and facilitates autolytic debridement • Its moisture retentive properties can enhance autolysis of eschar or drier wounds	Autolytic	• No absorption • Allows visualization of the wound • Can macerate periwound skin • Use caution on frail skin; adhesive can damage • If used as primary dressing, wound should have none or scant drainage • Use on intact skin for protection by decreasing friction • Can be used on dry eschar utilizing the moisture-retentive properties for autolytic debridement	• Prevention • Stage I or II • Primary or secondary dressing	3 x per week
Absorb exudate	Hydrocolloid Comfeel Restore DuoDERM Tegasorb	• Adhesive, occlusive, or semiocclusive dressings composed of various materials; carboxymethylcellulose, gelatin, and pectin • Absorbs light drainage • Can contain silver to assist with bacterial control • Promotes granulation, epithelialization, and facilitates autolytic debridement	Autolytic	• Can macerate periwound skin • May damage fragile periwound skin • Rolling and peeling of dressing can cause increased pressure and/or injury; try a larger size or different shape; can "melt out" along the edges	• Stage I, II • Shallow Stage III or IV	3 x per week
	Alginate Sorbsan CalciCare Kaltostat SeaSorb	• A seaweed-derived fiber of absorbent material, that reacts with wound fluid to form a gel • Absorbs moderate to high exudate rapidly • Can contain silver to assist with bacterial control • Has hemostatic properties • Promotes granulation, epithelialization, and facilitates autolytic debridement	Autolytic	• Requires secondary dressing • Not appropriate for dry wounds • Can be expensive for large wounds • Has hemostatic properties • Consider as an alternative to wet-to-dry dressing	• Exuding wounds	Daily
	Foams Allevyn Sof-Foam PolyMem Lyofoam Biatain	• Polyurethane hydrophilic semipermeable dressing • Promotes granulation and epithelialization • Absorbs moderate to high exudates, depending on the composition, generally not as quickly as alginates • Flexible and conforms to wound bed • Can contain silver to assist with bacterial control	Autolytic	• Available in adhesive and nonadhesive forms • May require secondary dressing if nonadhesive • Most have outside barrier layer • Usually slower absorption than alginates	• Stage I, II • Shallow Stage III or IV	3 x per week
	Wound fillers Multidex PolyWic Iodosorb Iodoflex FlexiGel Strands	• Absorbent, conformable filler available in beads, paste, powders, foams, and pillows • Highly absorbent, nonadherent. May include time-released antimicrobial to assist in the control of the bacterial load • Promotes granulation and epithelialization and facilitates autolytic debridement • Soft and moldable, therefore not causing any pressure inside the wound, especially when patient sits up in a chair • Absorption depends on product composition	Autolytic	• Require secondary dressing • Some products expand with absorption, fill only half full to avoid leakage out of wound • Brands that are applied wet can be used on low-exudate wounds to maintain a moist environment • Enhances microenvironment in cavity wounds, especially with uneven wound beds • Some are good inexpensive alternatives • Alternative for wet-to-dry dressings in larger wounds	• Wounds with depth	Need to check individual product due to variety in this category
Enzymatic debridement	Collagenase Papain-urea	• Active enzyme to destroy necrotic tissue from a wound bed • Enzyme stays active for 24 hours: daily wound care • Ointment base to provide vehicle and keeps wound bed moist • Selective to nonviable tissue	Enzymatic	• Requires secondary dressing • Can dry a shallow wound; avoid by adjusting secondary dressing • Papain urea may cause stinging in some wounds • Large amounts of necrotic tissue still need sharp debridement	• Necrotic wounds	Prescription required

*Semipermeable: allows transmission of moisture vapor from wound bed and inflow of oxygen; it is impermeable to water, stool, and bacteria.
**TAD: Transparent Adhesive Dressing
Note: The characteristics are indicative for most dressings in the generic category; there are many dressings that possess various combinations of properties.
Copyright Stoia Bales Consultants, 2003. Reprinted with permission.

other ways to decrease the bacteria count. As mentioned before, cleansing with volume, regardless of solution, may be all that is needed. Consider a cadexomer iodine if the burden needs to be controlled. The risks and benefits need to be considered.

Advantages

- Variable organism coverage
- Solutions usually readily available

Disadvantages

- Short half-life
- Cytotoxicity
- Slower healing

Product Examples

Acetic acid	Prepared by local pharmacy but available from several sources
Sodium hypochlorites (Dakin's® solution)	Prepared by local pharmacy but available from several sources
Hydrogen peroxide	Generic
Cadexomer iodine	Healthpoint Medical
Providone-iodine	Generic

ALGINATES

Action

Alginates are derived from brown seaweed and composed of soft, nonwoven fibers shaped as pads (fibrous mats) or ropes (twisted fibers). They are absorbent and conform to the shape of the wound. When packed into the wound, the alginate comes in contact with the wound exudate, forming a soft gel that maintains moist wound healing principles. Calcium alginates can also be used for their thrombogenic properties on wounds that are friable.

FIGURE 10-10
Calcium Alginates

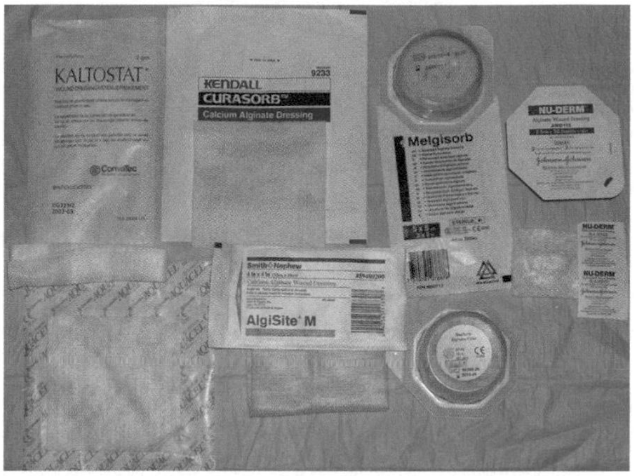

Indications

Alginates are used on partial- and full-thickness wounds with moderate to heavy exudate. They can be used with

- tunneling wounds
- infected and noninfected wounds
- sinus tracts
- wounds with necrotic debris
- moist, yellow, or red wounds.

Advantages

- Absorb up to 20 times their weight in exudate
- Fill in dead space
- Easy to apply and remove
- Facilitate autolytic debridement
- Help control odor

Disadvantages

- Contraindicated for wounds that have light exudate or dry eschar and dehydrated wounds
- Require a secondary dressing

Product Examples

Tegagen™ HI and Tegagen™ HG	3M Health Care
AlgiSite M	Smith & Nephew, Inc.
CarraSorb™ H	Carrington Laboratories, Inc.
SeaSorb™	Coloplast Corp.
Kaltostat®	ConvaTec

Restore CalciCare™   Hollister, Inc.

Sorbsan®   Bertek Pharmaceuticals, Inc.

BIOSYNTHETICS

Action

Biosynthetics were developed as temporary coverage for burn wounds, but their usage has since evolved into either short- or long-term use on multiple wounds involving skin loss, such as skin tears and donor sites. Biosynthetic dressings can be either a gel or a semiocclusive sheet and may require some form of freezing. Biosynthetic dressings foster healing by reepithelialization.

Indications

Biosynthetic dressings are used as primary dressings for wounds with skin loss and minimal to moderate drainage, such as

- skin tears
- donor sites
- abrasions
- burns
- chronic ulcers
- pressure ulcers.

Advantages

- Can be left in place for up to 10 days
- Nonadherent

Disadvantages

- Contraindicated for infected wounds
- Contraindicated for heavily draining wounds
- Expensive

Product Examples

AlloDerm   LifeCell Corp.

Biobrane®   Bertek Pharmaceuticals, Inc.

Hyalofill® Biopolymeric   ConvaTec

Oasis®   Healthpoint Medical

ANTIMICROBIALS

This section is divided into two categories; antimicrobial/antifungal topicals and antimicrobial dressings. The action of the product depends upon whether it is an antimicrobial, antifungal, or an antibiotic product. Each product differs slightly in its indication as well as its advantages and disadvantages to the specific therapy. The information presented here is not all-inclusive. It is important to read the product literature for each preparation or consult a pharmaceutical reference. In general, these agents are utilized to decrease the topical load of bacteria or contaminants found in the wound bed or on the surrounding skin. By lowering the number of bacteria on the surface, thereby reducing the bacterial load, the agent assists in reducing colonization and decreases the risk of infection. Many times, adequate cleansing and debridement are sufficient to dilute the number of bacteria. Bacterial contamination is usually associated with necrotic tissue within the wound bed. The quickest way to decrease that contamination is to rid the wound of necrotic tissue by debridement. If debridement is not indicated, thorough irrigation can assist in reducing the bacterial load. The *AHCPR Clinical Practice Guidelines* recommend that if a clean wound is not healing or continues to have exudate despite optimal care for 2–4 weeks, the clinician should consider a 2-week trial of topical antibiotics that are effective against gram-negative, gram-positive, and anaerobic organisms (for example, sulfadiazine, or triple antibiotics). These products should not be used for extended periods because of the increased chance of sensitivity, resistance, and secondary infection. Some products require a prescription and others may be obtained over-the-counter. The clinician must ensure a moist wound environment that is normally achieved by the occlusive nature of the ointment base.

ANTIMICROBIAL/ANTIFUNGAL TOPICALS

Antimicrobial/antifungal topicals are available in cream, ointment, lotion, spray, and powder forms, which are topically applied to the skin or wound. Some formulations also function as a moisture barrier ointment; usually these formulations have an antifungal agent present. The use of topical antibiotics has been a long-standing controversy, particularly because they are often used too liberally and for long periods. This raises concerns over the development of antimicrobial resistance, contact dermatitis, and sensitization.

Action

The majority of antimicrobial/antifungal topicals act on the cell membrane by either affecting the membrane's permeability or its synthesis. Antifungal agents vary in dosing but are generally recommended twice a day for 2–4 weeks. Relief of symptoms should begin within 24–48 hours with clinical improvement in 1 week; it is important to continue treatment for 2–4 weeks to achieve resolution. Antibiotics usually require more frequent application (2–6 times daily); this may vary according to the indication (either treatment of infection or reduction of bacterial load).

Indications

Antimicrobial/antifungal topicals are indicated for fungal, yeast, and bacterial infections that are diagnosed or strongly suspected. Yeast is commonly treated emperically; definitive diagnosis can be confirmed by potassium hydroxide (KOH) stain. Judicious prophylactic use may be indicated if the risk of infection is increased due to invasive procedures, viral or metabolic diseases, chemotherapy, radiotherapy, prolonged corticosteroid therapy, or environmental exposure, such as from diarrhea (Motta, 2003).

Advantages

- Available in various forms
- Readily available and available in generic forms. Most are inexpensive.
- Can be used with a variety of secondary dressings

Disadvantages

- Contraindicated with sensitivity to the agent or the vehicle
- Require prescription for some agents
- Frequent applications for some agents
- Use of neomycin causes a greater incidence of allergic sensitivity and cross-sensitivity to other aminoglycosides than other topical antibiotics, especially in wounds because they have lost their epidermal barrier (Sussman & Bates-Jensen, 2004)
- Clinicians tend to use antibiotics

Product Examples (Prescription)

Nitrofurazone (Furacin)	Norwich Eaton Pharmaceuticals, Inc.
Gentamicin ointment	Geneva Pharmaceuticals, Inc.
Ketoconazole (Nizoral)	Janssen Pharmaceuticals
Lotrimin cream (antifungal)	Schering-Plough
Metronidazole (MetroGel)	Curatek Pharmaceuticals, Inc.
Mupirocin (Bactroban) ointment	GlaxoSmithKline
Nystatin cream/ powder (antifungal)	Rugby Pharmaceuticals
Silver sulfadiazine cream (Thermazene)	Kendall Healthcare
Silver sulfadiazine cream (Silvadene)	Marion Merrell Dow
Sulfamylon® solution & cream	Bertek Pharmaceuticals

Product Examples (Non-Prescription)

Aloe Vesta® antifungal ointment	ConvaTec
Carrington® antifungal cream	Carrington Laboratories, Inc.
Biafine	Medix Pharmaceuticals Americas, Inc.
Bacitracin ointment	Parmed Pharmaceuticals
Baza® cream (antifungal)	Coloplast Corp.
Mitrazol™ cream/ powder (antifungal)	Healthpoint Medical
Mycostatin cream/ powder (antifungal)	Westwood-Squibb Pharmaceuticals, Inc.
Neosporin sulfate (Neosporin)	Pfizer
Polysporin ointment	Pfizer
Tinactin (antifungal)	Schering-Plough

ANTIMICROBIAL DRESSINGS
Action

Antimicrobial dressings deliver the effects of such agents as silver and polyhexamethylene biguanide (PHMB), to maintain efficacy against common infectious bacteria (Motta, 2003). Silver inhibits respiratory enzyme function of bacterial cells but not human cells. Silver has a long history in health care. It was first used in 1834 by Credé as 1% silver nitrate, which was placed into the eyes of newborns to prevent blindness from infection. The U.S. FDA approved silver solutions for use in wounds in the 1920s. The burn community used silver solution with high dressing change frequency because of the short duration of the product. Silver solution was shown to improve wound healing, possibly by anti-inflammatory mechanisms (Warriner, 2002). Silver sulfadiazine cream became the silver dressing of choice because it could be applied 1–2 times per day. The newer silver dressings are silver-coated polymeric substrates that are applied directly to the wound surface. Their effectiveness is based on the biological activity of silver. Different forms are available: silver-coated sheets and fabrics; powders; and silver imbedded in alginate, hydrocolloid, and foam dressings. The silver remains active from 3–7 days, making these dressings a welcome addition to the chronic wound community. Silver protects against a broad spectrum of organisms, including MRSA, VRE, yeasts, and molds. These products are effective and useful in many situations but should never be used as substitutes for systemic antibiotics in the case of invasive soft tissue infection.

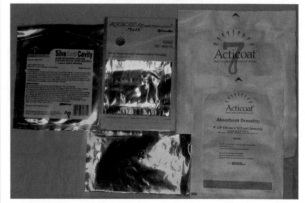

FIGURE 10-11
Silver Products

Advantages

- Duration of antimicrobial activity
- Broad coverage
- Available in various modalities

Disadvantages

- Expensive
- Some need moistening with water to activate
- Silver staining with some dressings
- Certain products need secondary dressings

Product Examples

Biopatch™	Johnson & Johnson Wound Management Worldwide
Acticoat	Smith & Nephew, Inc.
Arglaes™	Medline Industries, Inc.
Calgitrol Ag/Ag Plus	Magnus Bio-Medical Technologies, Inc.

Island Wound Dressing   Medwrap Corp.
with Microban

Kerlix® AMD Roll/   Kendall
Super Sponge

Silverlon™   Argentum Medical LLC

Silveron™   Silveron Consumer
                          Products

COLLAGENS

Action

Collagen is an insoluble, fibrous protein that is produced by fibroblasts. Its fibers are found in connective tissues, such as bone, skin, ligaments, and cartilage. Collagen dressings may encourage the deposition and organization of new collagen fibers as well as encourage new development of granulation tissue. They are also thought to stimulate new tissue growth and wound debridement. Collagen dressings are made as sheets, pads, particles, and gels. These products absorb exudate, maintain moist wound healing, conform to the wound surface, are nonadherent, and can be used with other topical agents.

Indications

Collagen dressings can be used as a primary dressing for

- wounds with minimal to moderate exudate
- infected and noninfected wounds
- tunneling wounds
- skin grafts
- red or yellow wounds
- donor sites.

Advantages

- Nonadherent
- Easy to apply and remove
- Can be used in combination with other topical agents

Disadvantages

- Require a secondary dressing
- May not be recommended for full-thickness burns or black wounds
- May cause allergic reactions for patients with a sensitivity to biomaterial sources, such as bovine, porcine, or avian

Product Examples

Fibracol™ Collagen   Johnson & Johnson
Alginate   Wound Management
                         Worldwide

Medifil Gel   BioCore Medical
                         Technologies, Inc.

Promogran Matrix   Johnson & Johnson
                         Wound Management
                         Worldwide

COMPOSITES

Action

Composite dressings are a combination of two or more products that have moisture-retentive properties as well as absorptive properties. To be classified as a composite dressing, the dressing must have the following features: a bacterial barrier, an absorptive layer, a semiadherent or nonadherent property for covering the wound bed, and an adhesive border.

FIGURE 10-12
Composites

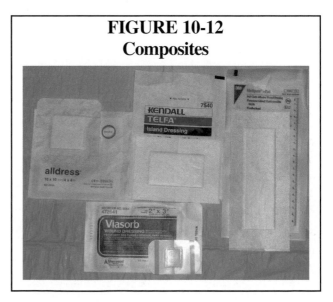

Composite dressings may assist with autolytic debridement, allow for exchange of moisture vapor, and conform well to the wound shape.

Indications

Composite dressings are used on partial- to full-thickness wounds with moderate to heavy exudate. They can be used with

- a healthy wound bed
- necrotic tissue
- mixture of granulation and necrotic tissue.

Composite dressings may be used as either primary or secondary dressings.

Advantages

- Easy to apply and remove
- May be used on infected wounds

Product Examples

Alldress® Care	Molnlycke Health
Covaderm Plus®	DeRoyal Wound Care
OpSite Post-Op	Smith & Nephew, Inc.
Primapore	Smith & Nephew, Inc.
Telfa® Plus	Kendall
CombiDerm®	ConvaTec
Medipore™	3M Health Care

FOAMS

Action

Foam dressings are semipermeable and either hydrophilic or hydrophobic. They are nonlinting, are absorbent, and vary in thickness. They have a nonadherent contact layer that provides for nontraumatic removal. Foam dressings help create a moist environment and provide thermal insulation to the wound. Certain foam dressings have an adhesive border and may also contain a film coating as an additional barrier to bacterial invasion. Foam dressings come as pads, sheets, and cavity fillers.

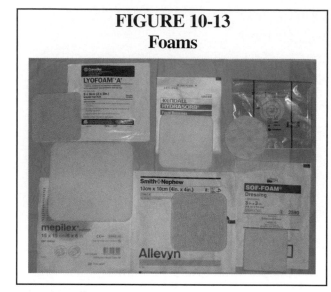

FIGURE 10-13
Foams

Indications

Foam dressings are used in both partial- and full-thickness wounds with minimal, moderate, or heavy drainage. They can be used as primary coverings to provide absorption or insulation or as secondary dressings for wounds that need packing or additional absorption. Foam dressings are also indicated for controlling drainage from around tube sites. They have been used extensively under compression wraps in the treatment of venous ulcers.

Advantages

- Easy to apply and remove
- May be used under compression
- Absorb moderate to heavy exudate
- Can repel contaminents
- Nonadherent forms do not injure surrounding skin
- Flexible

Disadvantages

- Not recommended for dry eschar or wounds with no exudate
- May require a secondary dressing, such as netting or tape, for securing to the skin
- May macerate the skin if they become saturated

Product Examples

Allevyn	Smith & Nephew, Inc.
Biatain™	Coloplast Corp.
Curafoam®	Kendall
HydroCell Foam	Dumex Medical
Lyofoam®	ConvaTec
NU-DERM	Johnson & Johnson Wound Management Worldwide
PolyMem®	Ferris Manufacturing Corp.
Sof-Foam™	Johnson & Johnson Wound Management Worldwide
Tielle™	Johnson & Johnson Wound Management Worldwide

GAUZES (WOVEN AND NONWOVEN)

Action

Gauze dressings are manufactured in many forms, including impregnated, woven or nonwoven, fine meshed, or open coarser mesh. Fabric composition may include cotton, polyester, or rayon. They are available sterile or nonsterile in various sizes: pads, rolls, or packing strips. They may be used as primary or secondary dressings and as a form of mechanical debridement with wet-to-dry dressing changes. Gauze dressings may act as moisture-retentive dressings when applied as either wet-to-moist or damp dressings. They may also be used dry.

Gauze dressings are classified as moderately absorptive, cost-effective, and readily available. The cost effectiveness varies depending on the frequency of dressing change. When dressings are every 4–6 hours and staff time is calculated, these products can be more expensive than other products requiring less frequent dressing changes. They can be combined with topical agents or with other types of dressings. Gauze dressings can be packed into tunnels or areas of dead space and "fluffed" for added absorption capability. When used for packing, gauze dressings should not be packed so tightly that they impede blood flow.

Indications

Dry gauze dressings are used primarily to protect the wound bed from trauma and infection as well as to wick exudate away from the wound area. Sterile gauze is used after sharp debridement. Moist gauze dressings are used to facilitate a moist wound environment for healing. They are cost-effective when used on large cavity wounds. The gauze may be moistened with a solution or impregnated with a medication. Some fine mesh gauze may be impregnated with an ointment to prevent dryness of the wound bed without allowing maceration. Wet-to-dry gauze dressings are used for mechanical debridement. Gauze dressings can be used as either primary or secondary dressings.

GAUZES — ALL PURPOSE, PACKING, AND DEBRIDING

Advantages

- Readily available
- Can be cost effective depending on use
- Moderately absorptive
- Can be used with other topical preparations
- Can be packed or fluffed into tunneling wounds
- Can maintain moisture over a longer period of time (impregnated gauze)
- Can be used over shallow wounds or with medication, preventing drying out of the wound bed or ineffective medication (impregnated gauze)

Disadvantages

- May require frequent changes
- May be painful with dressing removal
- May easily show strike-through or leakage
- May adhere to the wound and traumatize healthy tissue

Product Examples

CURITY®	Kendall
KERLIX®	Kendall
MIRASORB	Johnson & Johnson Sponges Medical, Inc.

GAUZES — IMPREGNATED

Advantages

- Readily available
- Can be cost effective depending on use
- Can be used with other topical preparations or dressings
- Assist in keeping the wound bed moist
- Assist with autolytic debridement
- Can be used as a wound contact layer (coarse mesh)

Disadvantages

- May macerate the surrounding skin if excess drainage is present
- Usually more expensive than dry gauze
- Used most often on superficial wounds
- May cause allergies depending on the type

Product Examples

Adaptic™	Johnson & Johnson
Aquaphor	Smith & Nephew, Inc.
Curasalt	Kendall
Dermagran®	Derma Sciences, Inc.
Mesalt®	Molnlycke Health Care
Scarlet Red	Kendall
Gelocast®	BSN/Jobst
Vaseline®	Kendall
Xeroform	Kendall

GAUZES — NONADHERENT

Advantages

- Keep dressing from sticking to the wound bed and disrupting granulation tissue
- Can have an absorptive layer
- Readily available
- Inexpensive
- Can be used with other topical preparations

Disadvantages

- Not absorptive
- May macerate the surrounding skin (most do not allow exudate flow through dressing)
- Can adhere to the wound bed on removal
- May require frequent dressing changes

Product Examples

Adaptic	Johnson & Johnson
Telfa®	Kendall

GAUZES — WRAPPING

Product Examples

Conform®	Kendall
Durlix	Dumex Medical
Kerlix®	Kendall
KLING Fluff Rolls	Johnson & Johnson

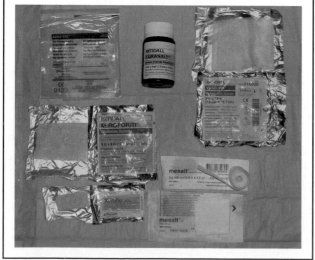

FIGURE 10-14
Impregnated Gauze

HYDROCOLLOIDS

Action

Hydrocolloids are occlusive or semiocclusive wound care products comprised of several hydroactive materials, including gelatin, pectin, and carboxymethylcellulose. The hydroactive material interacts with moisture from the wound bed to form a moist environment over the wound. The composition of the layer that comes in contact with the wound bed may vary considerably among the hydrocolloids. The thickness and composition of the product determines its absorptive capability. These dressings provide a moist healing environment that allows granulation of clean wounds and autolytic debridement of necrotic wounds. Hydrocolloids commonly have an odor when they are removed. Pectin can contribute to the odor caused by the anaerobic environment. A few of the hydrocolloid dressings leave a residue in the wound. This is not a cause for alarm and can be easily removed during the cleaning process.

Hydrocolloid dressings come in different forms. The most common is the wafer, which comes in various thicknesses, shapes, and sizes. Studies have shown that the shape designed for the sacral area increases the weartime of the dressing. There are also shapes designed for the heel to create a friend-lier application process. Other forms of hydrocolloids are pastes and powders. These forms are usually used to fill in dead space of an uneven wound bed.

Indications

Hydrocolloid dressings are used on
- partial-thickness or superficial full-thickness wounds
- wounds with or without necrotic debris
- wounds with light to moderate drainage.

These dressings can be utilized as either a primary or secondary dressings.

Advantages
- Facilitate autolytic debridement
- Impermeable to bacteria and other contaminants
- Permeable to moisture vapor but not water
- Self-adhesive
- Mold well
- Provide light to moderate exudate absorption
- Can be left in place for 3–5 days
- May be used under compression
- Available in thick or thin versions to accommodate varying amounts of exudate
- Some brands allow visualization of the wound bed through the dressing

Disadvantages
- Edges may roll or "melt out"
- May tear surrounding skin on removal
- Not recommended for wounds with heavy exudate, tunneling, or infections or with bone or other exposed structures
- Most are not transparent, which diminishes evaluation potential and results in early removal of dressing
- Limit gas exchange between the wound and the environment (occlusive dressings)
- Cause formation of hypergranulation tissue on the wound bed
- May macerate the immediate periwound skin

FIGURE 10-15
Hydrocolloids

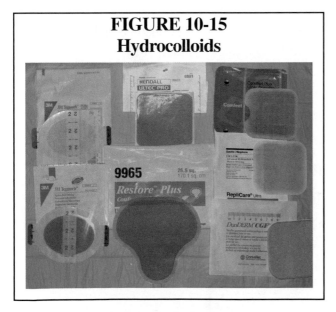

Product Examples

3M Tegasorb™	3M Health Care
CarraSmart™	Carrington Laboratories, Inc.
Comfeel®	Coloplast Corp.
Cutinova	Smith & Nephew, Inc.
DuoDERM®	ConvaTec
Exuderm	Medline Industries, Inc
Hydrocol®	Bertek Pharmaceuticals
PrimaCol	Dumex
RepliCare®	Smith & Nephew, Inc.
Restore™	Hollister, Inc.
Ultec®	Kendall

HYDROGELS

Action

Hydrogels are nonadherent dressings composed of water, polymers, glycerin, and other ingredients that create an amorphous gel or gel sheet. The amorphous gels are packaged in tubes and impregnated gauzes. They are designed to donate moisture to a dry wound or maintain the moisture of a moist wound bed. This facilitates autolytic debridement and promotes granulation tissue and epithelialization. Due to their high water content, they are not used for wounds that have a high amount of exu-

---

date. Conversely, the high water content can allow drying of the wound bed on superficial wounds. To prevent drying, a secondary dressing, which assists in the retention of moisture, may be helpful. An ointment-impregnated gauze, like Adaptic or Vaseline gauze, may also be helpful . Hydrogels also have the ability to cool the wound; the cooling effect decreases discomfort in painful wounds.

Indications

Hydrogel dressings may be used with either partial- or full-thickness wounds. They may be used for

* clean, granulating acute and chronic wounds with mild exudate
* necrotic or sloughing wounds
* minor burns
* wounds caused by radiation.

Advantages

* Facilitate autolytic debridement, granulation, and epithelialization
* Fill in dead space
* Rehydrate the wound bed
* Soothe and reduces pain
* Easy to apply and remove
* Can be used with infected wounds

Disadvantages

* Provide minimal absorption of exudate
* Cannot be used with moderate to heavy exudate
* Usually require secondary dressings
* When product has high water content, may dry out on superficial wounds
* May be difficult to secure
* May cause maceration of periwound skin
* May not keep out bacteria if used alone

Product Examples

Tegagel™	3M Health Care
Carrasyn®	Carrington Laboratories, Inc.
Comfeel®	Coloplast Corp.
Curasol™	Healthpoint

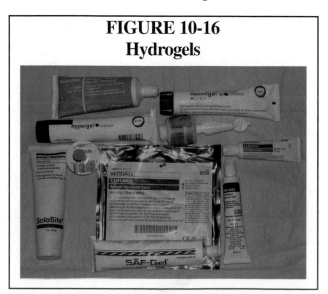

FIGURE 10-16
Hydrogels

Hypergel®	Molnlycke
IntraSite	Smith & Nephew, Inc.
Nu-Gel	Johnson & Johnson Medical Inc.
Restore™	Hollister, Inc.
Saf-Gel™	ConvaTec
Skintegrity™	Medline Industries, Inc.

MOISTURE BARRIER PREPARATIONS

This category includes ointments, creams, emollients, and skin pastes that are used on partial-thickness injuries in the presence of diarrhea or wound exudate. When irritation occurs, protect the skin from further injury by promoting healing and decreasing pain. Moisture barriers repel liquid and can be applied to the skin along with any nonadhere dressing. They are a supplement to primary wound care. In the perineal area, the barrier cream or ointment can be utilized as a primary dressing to avoid the difficulty of keeping a dressing in place or soiling from incontinence. When the skin is weepy, it is more difficult to apply the treatment. Several of the products listed here adhere slightly to wet skin, allowing protection needed to heal the area. These products can be utilized in the perineal area or on periwound skin. Remember the goal is to optimize skin by protecting it from injury and healing it.

Product Examples

Critic-Aid®	Coloplast Corp.
Calmoseptine	Calmoseptine, Inc.
Cavilon™ Durable Barrier Cream	3M Health Care
Desitin	Pfizer
A & D Ointment	Schering-Plough
Triple Care® Extra Protective Cream	Smith & Nephew, Inc.

SPECIALTY ABSORPTIVES

Action

Specialty absorptive dressings are multilayer products that provide such characteristics as a semi-adherent or nonadherent wound surface layer, combined with a highly absorptive layer of fibers comprised of either absorbent cellulose, cotton, or rayon. Specialty absorptive dressings may have an adhesive border or may require additional securing to the wound edges. They are usually available in larger sizes and a variety of shapes.

Indications

Specialty absorptive dressings can be used as either primary or secondary dressings to manage light to heavy exudate on surgical incisions, lacerations, burns, donor graft sites, or any acute or chronic exuding wound. They are appropriate with infected or noninfected wounds and with granulating or necrotic sloughing wounds.

Advantages

*   Easy to apply
*   Nonadherent, which minimizes trauma to tissues on removal
*   Absorbent
*   Can be used as secondary dressings over most primary dressings

Disadvantages

*   May not be appropriate as primary dressings for undermined wounds
*   Expensive for large sizes

Product Examples

Covaderm®	DeRoyal
Dupad Abdominal Pad	Dumex
Exu-Dry®	Smith & Nephew, Inc.
Intersorb®	Kendall
Mepore®	Molnlycke Health Care

TRANSPARENT FILMS

Action

Transparent film dressings are synthetic, adhesive, semipermeable, nonabsorptive, polyurethane membrane dressings that are manufactured in varying thicknesses and sizes. They are known by multiple names, including polyurethane film, moisture-vapor permeable dressing, transparent adhesive dressing (TAD), and the IV dressing. They are waterproof and impermeable to bacteria and contaminants, yet permit oxygen and water vapor to cross the barrier. The moisture vapor transmission rate, or the amount of moisture that can pass through the dressing, varies with the thickness and production of the dressing. Products with higher rates of transmission are usually marketed as IV dressings. Fluid that accumulates must pass through the surface; when this rate of accumulation surpasses the rate of vapor transmission, the fluid begins to pool under the dressing. It creates a pseudoblister, which can be left in place if the exudate is over the wound bed. Once the fluid flows onto the surrounding skin, the dressing should be changed to avoid maceration. The maintenance of a moist wound environment promotes granulation tissue formation and autolytic debridement of necrotic tissue. Because they are moisture retentive, these dressings can be used on dry eschar to begin the autolytic process. They enhance epithelial migration, resulting in faster healing and less scarring. The surface of the dressing reduces surface tension, thereby decreasing friction and shear to the skin. Their transparent nature also allows visualization of the wound bed. Dressings may be left in place for a week or more, depending on the wound type. The longer wear-time allows for easier and less traumatic dressing removal as the natural sloughing of skin occurs. The method of removal of TADs can minimize trauma to skin. The dressing should not be pulled back over itself. The film should be carefully pulled away from itself (parallel to the skin) while applying light pressure to the center of the dressing to minimize the pulling force until the entire dressing is removed.

Indications

Transparent film dressings are utilized as primary or secondary dressings for superficial partial-thickness wounds that have little to no exudate, with or without necrosis, including

- Stage I and II pressure ulcers
- Lacerations or abrasions
- Donor sites
- IV sites
- Prevention against injury to intact skin
- Dry eschar (for short term use to initiate autolytic debridement)

Advantages

- Have extended wear-time on nondraining or newly epithelized skin, thereby reducing nursing time and the likelihood of trauma to new tissue or fragile surrounding skin
- Retain moisture
- Flexible
- Facilitate autolytic debridement
- Impermeable to bacteria and other contaminants, therefore protecting from incontinence and other types of drainage
- Allow for visualization of the wound bed
- Do not require a secondary dressing
- Reduce trauma from shear and friction

Disadvantages

- May not be recommended for infected wounds
- May be difficult to apply
- May roll at the edges in high friction areas
- May loosen if exudate is too heavy
- Nonabsorptive
- Must be used cautiously with fragile peri-wound skin
- Require a border of intact dry skin for adhesive edge of dressing

Product Examples

Tegaderm™	3M Health Care
BlisterFilm®	Kendall
CarraSmart™	Carrington Laboratories, Inc.
OpSite	Smith & Nephew, Inc.

TOPICAL PREPARATIONS

WOUND FILLERS
Action

Wound fillers are produced in a variety of forms, including pastes, powders, beads, granules, and gels. Wound fillers usually provide a moist wound environment for healing, manage exudate, and help with autolytic debridement through the addition of moisture to necrotic tissue. They are nonadherant and require a secondary dressing. They are used to fill dead space. Consideration needs to be given to the patient's or caregiver's ability to remove or cleanse the dressing and also to cost when treating large wounds. If a wound is large, the wound filler can be used on the base of the wound and the wound filled with normal saline moistened gauze. Some products may include an antimicrobial that is time-released as exudate is absorbed into the dressing.

Indication

Wound fillers are used as primary dressings for wounds that are full thickness and have minimal to heavy exudate, are infected or noninfected, and require some form of packing in order to fill dead space (see Figures 2-4 & 10-8).

Advantages
- Fill in dead space
- Easy to apply and remove
- Absorb moderate to heavy exudate
- Facilitate autolytic debridement and rehydrate necrotic tissue
- Some may be used in conjunction with other products

- Conform to the wound bed
- Help with odor control

Disadvantages
- May dehydrate the wound depending on amount of exudate
- Require secondary dressing
- Are not recommended for wounds with light drainage or dry eschar
- May need to allow for expansion of the product due to the absorption of exudate
- Expensive with large wounds

Product Examples

Comfeel® Paste	Coloplast Corp.
Dermagran® Hydrophilic-B	Derma Sciences, Inc.
DuoDERM®	ConvaTec
FlexiGel® Strands	Smith & Nephew, Inc.
Iodosorb™ Gel	Healthpoint
Iodoflex™ Pad	Healthpoint
Multidex®	DeRoyal
Polywic®	Ferris Manufacturing Corp.

ENZYMATIC DEBRIDING AGENTS
Action

Enzymatic debriding agents are chemicals that work by digesting necrotic tissue. Different types of enzymes target different types of tissue: protein, fibrin, collagen. Enzymes are not active in a dry environment and, therefore, cannot be used on dry eschar unless the eschar is crosshatched and a moist environment is maintained. The main enzymatic debriding agents on the market at the time of this writing are collagenase and a papain-urea combination. Papain is the enzyme but urea is needed to activate this enzyme. The presence of some heavy metals, salts, antimicrobials, and wound cleansers can inactivate the enzymes, so they should be avoided. Enzymes are generally applied once a day, the length of time the enzyme remains active in its preparation. If drainage increases due to the liquefaction of necrotic tissue, a different secondary dressing may be chosen or dressing change frequency can be increased to twice a day, but cost should be considered.

Indication

Enzymatic debriding agents are indicated for the debridement of necrotic tissue in acute or chronic wounds, such as pressure ulcers, neuropathic ulcers, traumatic wounds, surgical wounds, and burns. Enzymes are useful on moist wounds with moderate amounts of necrotic tissue. They are used when a patient is not a candidate for or the setting is not conducive to surgery or sharp debridement. These agents should be discontinued after a clean wound bed is established.

Advantages

• Easy to apply and remove (no special training needed)

• Promote selective debridement

• Require once-a-day application

Disadvantages

• Require hard eschar to be scored or cross-hatched

• Require a secondary dressing

• Require a prescription

• Slow form of debridement

Product Examples

Accuzyme® (papain-urea)	Healthpoint
Ethezyme (papain-urea)	Ethex
Gladase (papain-urea)	Smith & Nephew, Inc.
Panafil® (papain-urea)	Healthpoint Medical
Santyl (collagenase)	Smith & Nephew, Inc.

SUMMARY

With today's technology, the ability to manage a wound's microenvironment seems limitless. Hundreds of products are available to either help add moisture to the wound or absorb exudate from the wound. There are products that assist in the debridement of necrotic tissue, provide warmth and protection to the wound bed, and help to decrease the topical bacterial load in the wound bed. However, the myth still remains among clinicians and patients that products heal wounds. In reality, the complex management of wounds exists to provide the best environment for the body to heal the wound. Understanding the principles of managing a wound and its microenvironment, as well as understanding the different wound product classifications, helps the clinician choose the appropriate topical therapy to achieve the desired outcome. Selecting a wound dressing for a particular wound is a matter of matching the environment with the most appropriate dressing. The clinician must choose the best dressing to manage the exudate, while providing a moist wound environment and a dry periwound skin environment. Effective wound management involves constant reevaluation of the wound treatment and adjustments in topical wound care as needed. It also requires educational updates to remain abreast of the latest technological advancements. Even though topical treatment of the wound is at times critical in achieving the expected outcome, it is essential that the clinician also keeps in mind the fundamentals of wound healing and the multiple factors involved in the formation, treatment, and resolution of a wound.

EXAM QUESTIONS

CHAPTER 10
Questions 77-90

77. The known impediments to wound repair are

    a. infection, necrotic tissue, and pooled exudate.

    b. infection, ischemic tissue, and beefy granulation.

    c. slough, eschar, and beefy granulation.

    d. eschar, pus, and epithelial ridge.

78. Colonization can be described as

    a. local infection with cellulitis.

    b. high bioburden on the wound surface.

    c. a wound showing signs of deterioration.

    d. low bacterial count on a wound surface.

79. A contributing factor that adds to the development of infection is

    a. foul odor of wound exudate.

    b. creamy exudate from a wound.

    c. impairment or lack of blood flow to the area.

    d. the use of occlusive dressings.

80. The culture method that would give the truest picture of a pathogen causing a wound infection is a

    a. swab culture.

    b. needle aspirate.

    c. curettage of the wound base.

    d. tissue biopsy.

81. According to the *AHCPR Clinical Practice Guidelines*, the range of irrigation pressures that is considered safe and effective is

    a. 10–15 psi.

    b. 4–15 psi.

    c. 2–20 psi.

    d. 6–8 psi.

82. When treating a clean granulating wound, the cleansing solution of choice would be

    a. an antiseptic.

    b. sterile water.

    c. normal saline solution.

    d. hydrogen peroxide.

83. The quickest method of debridement is

    a. mechanical.

    b. sharp.

    c. chemical.

    d. autolytic.

84. The methods that are considered types of mechanical debridement are

    a. whirlpool, pulse lavage, scrubbing, wet-to-dry dressing, and irrigation.

    b. whirlpool, pulse lavage, use of enzymes, and irrigation.

    c. irrigation, whirlpool, and drying the wound.

    d. autolysis, pulse lavage, scrubbing, wet-to-dry dressing, and irrigation.

85. Considerations that assist in the choice of debridement method for a patient are

    a. insurance coverage, product marketing brochure, and availability of method.

    b. patient setting, condition of the patient, and time available to staff.

    c. finances, reimbursement, and product marketing brochure.

    d. type of wound, finances, ability of the caregiver, and availability of methods.

86. The primary purpose of the wound dressing is to

    a. keep the wound bed moist and the surrounding skin dry.

    b. protect the wound from infection and contaminants.

    c. decrease the amount of contaminants and debris.

    d. promote granulation tissue.

87. Topical therapy enhances autolysis of nonviable tissue and

    a. decreases the amount of exudate and odor.

    b. increases erythema in the surrounding skin.

    c. increases the amount of exudate and mimics the appearance of pus.

    d. decreases induration around the wound.

88. An example of a periwound injury is

    a. skin rash.

    b. periwound induration.

    c. skin infection.

    d. maceration.

89. The dressings that provide an environment for autolytic debridement are

    a. alginates, wet-to-dry, and transparent films.

    b. alginates, hydrocolloids, and enzymes.

    c. enzymes, hydrocolloids, and transparent films.

    d. alginates, hydrocolloids, and transparent films.

90. Which of the following statements is true regarding topical antibiotic therapy?

    a. A 2-week trial is recommended on necrotic wounds that are nonhealing and continue to have exudate after 2-4 weeks of optimal care.

    b. It is useful in treating systemic infection.

    c. A 2-week trial is recommended on clean wounds that are nonhealing and continue to have exudate after 2–4 weeks of optimal care.

    d. It should be used on contaminated wounds.

CHAPTER 11

THE ART OF THE DRESSING CHANGE

CHAPTER OBJECTIVE

Upon completion of this chapter, the reader will be able to discuss how a wound dressing is removed, applied, and packed in a manner that is least detrimental to the patient. The reader will also be able to discuss the controversy over clean versus sterile technique in changing a wound.

LEARNING OBJECTIVES

Upon completion of the chapter, the reader will be able to

1. identify two aspects of dressing removal that help to protect periwound skin and the wound base.

2. describe two principles involved in packing a wound.

3. describe three options for securing a dressing.

4. state two options used to decrease pain associated with dressing change.

5. discuss the status of the current literature on the use of clean versus sterile technique in dressing change.

INTRODUCTION

The art of changing a wound dressing may seem as if it does not require any special skill, on the contrary, however, several important principles relate to the procedure of changing a dressing.

These principles maintain importance no matter what type of wound is being treated or what type of dressing is being used. In response to previous requests to provide information on general dressing changes, this chapter focuses on the principles associated with dressing removal, dressing application, packing wounds, securing the dressing, and pain management. A discussion on the use of clean versus sterile technique with dressing changes is also addressed, because this issue has been controversial in wound care management.

THE ART OF DRESSING REMOVAL

The wound dressing should be changed depending on several factors, such as type of wound, amount of drainage, type of dressing being used, availability of a caregiver, and financial considerations. Certain dressings, such as transparent dressings, have suggested methods of removal that the clinician should be aware of. The manufacturer usually lists on the product information any special methods of application or removal that are recommended for a particular product. Some general principles of dressing removal for all dressings include protecting the periwound skin and the wound bed from trauma. Adhesives should be removed in the direction of the hair growth, special adhesive removers may aid in their removal. Gauze that is moistened can be used to support the skin in the dressing removal process to avoid skin stripping (Bryant, 2000).

The dressing removal process is started by gently lifting or rolling one edge of the dressing with one hand and supporting the tissue that is adjacent to the dressing with the other hand or with moistened gauze. If any portion of the dressing is attached to or adheres to the wound bed, normal saline solution or wound cleanser may be used to moisten the dressing material and release the attached tissue before the dressing is gently removed. If the patient can shower and there are no contraindications to showering or getting the dressing wet, the shower may be an effective method of loosening the dressing to minimize any discomfort or damage in the removal process. It is important to read your facility's policy on dressing changes to note when gloves are changed and hands are washed or sanitized. The use of universal precautions should always be implemented with any dressing removal (Bryant, 2000). (See Figures 11-1 & 11-2.)

FIGURE 11-1
Dressing Removal 1

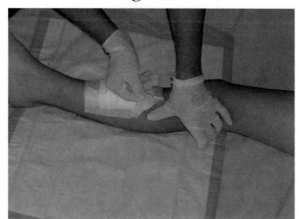

Gently lift the dressing on one corner with one hand while supporting the tissue adjacent to the dressing with the other hand.

FIGURE 11-2
Dressing Removal 2

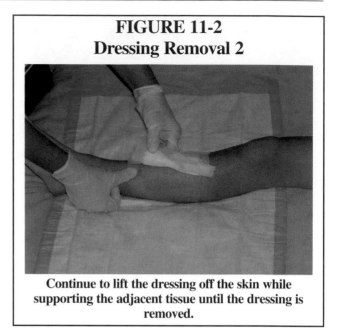

Continue to lift the dressing off the skin while supporting the adjacent tissue until the dressing is removed.

Disposal of the contaminated dressing depends on the clinical setting, infectious disease policies, type of organisms, and the amount of blood or drainage on the dressing. Acute, outpatient, and long-term care settings usually have specific infection control guidelines to follow for dressing disposal. Excessive amounts of blood or drainage may be handled in a special infectious waste bag. Wound infection with specific bacteria such as MRSA and VRE may require contact isolation precautions that would dictate the disposal of the dressing in an infectious waste bag. The policies in a home setting may be as stringent as in other settings. Dressings commonly are disposed of in the general refuse collection system; however, it is important to know the infection control guidelines for the clinical setting in which the dressing is being changed. With any dressing disposal, the use of universal precautions for blood and body fluids is mandatory.

THE ART OF DRESSING APPLICATION

The application of a wound dressing depends on the type of dressing that is used. Once again, many dressings have specific instructions from the manufacturer for application. The clinician should be aware of these instructions in order to obtain the best results from a particular dressing. Once the old dressing has been removed and the wound cleansed, the new dressing is applied with attention to peri-wound skin protection. A skin sealant can be applied to the periwound area prior to dressing application to protect the skin from irritation. When the skin sealant has dried, the wound dressing can be applied. Difficult to dress areas, such as heels, elbows, gluteal folds, and the gluteal cleft, may require dressing adjustments, such as trimming or molding, in order to obtain a good fit (Bryant, 2000). (See Figures 11-3 through 11-6.)

FIGURE 11-3
Dressing Application 1

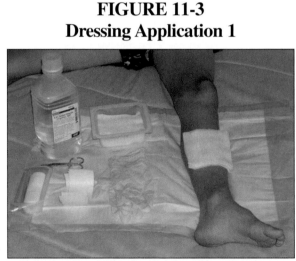

Prepare all supplies for the dressing change on a clean surface. Place the new dressing over the cleaned wound.

FIGURE 11-4
Dressing Application 2

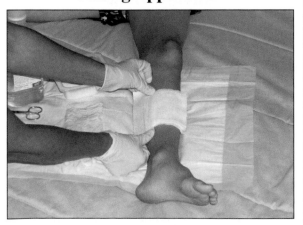

Apply tape to the dressing to secure it in place.

FIGURE 11-5
Dressing Application 3

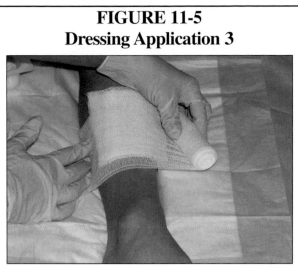

The dressing may also be applied using conform or a kerlix type roll.

FIGURE 11-6
Dressing Application 4

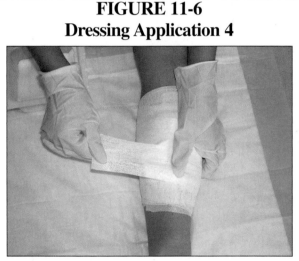

Secure the conform roll with tape after the roll has covered the dressing.

PACKING A WOUND

If the wound has some depth, tunneling, or under-mining, this dead space needs to be packed. Packing of dead space decreases the chance of abscess formation and assists in wound healing from the base upward to prevent premature contrac-tion and closure of the wound margins. Packing materials should be able to conform to the wound contours. The procedure for packing a wound includes a thorough assessment of the wound for depth. If any tunneling is noted, a packing material, such as strip gauze or strips of other wound dressings, are placed into the tunnel with a cotton-tipped applicator to allow for wicking of exudate and to fill in dead space. A tail of the packing strip should be left out of the wound for easy retrieval. For larger areas of depth or undermining, a variety of packing materials may be used, including absorbent impregnated gauze or fluffed gauze that is loosely placed into the wound. Additional gauze dressings or a secondary cover dressing can be used to further absorb exudate and to assist in securing the packing. Overpacking the wound should be avoided to decrease any delay in wound closure (Bryant, 2000). (See Figures 11-7 through 11-15.)

FIGURE 11-7
Packing Supplies

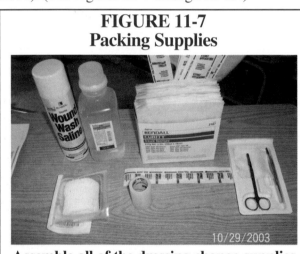

Assemble all of the dressing change supplies on a clean surface.

Photograph provided by Vivian Sternweiler, MS, RN, CWCN. Reprinted with permission.

FIGURE 11-8
Packing Procedure 1

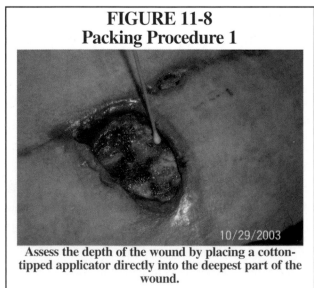

Assess the depth of the wound by placing a cotton-tipped applicator directly into the deepest part of the wound.

Photograph provided by Vivian Sternweiler, MS, RN, CWCN. Reprinted with permission.

FIGURE 11-9
Packing Procedure 2

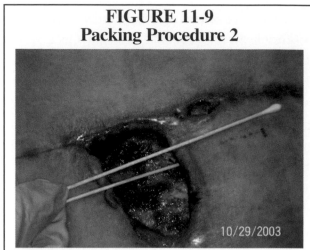

Assess for any undermining or tunneling of wound margins by gently probing with a cotton-tipped applicator.

Photograph provided by Vivian Sternweiler, MS, RN, CWCN. Reprinted with permission.

FIGURE 11-10
Packing Procedure 3

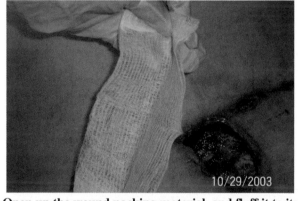

Open up the wound packing material, and fluff it to its largest capacity if gauze is being used as the packing material.

Photograph provided by Vivian Sternweiler, MS, RN, CWCN. Reprinted with permission.

FIGURE 11-11
Packing Procedure 4

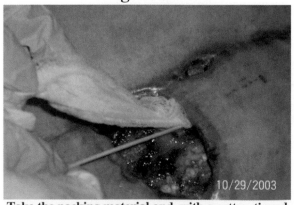

Take the packing material and, with a cotton-tipped applicator fill in the undermined or tunneled areas of the wound first.

Photograph provided by Vivian Sternweiler, MS, RN, CWCN. Reprinted with permission.

FIGURE 11-12
Packing Procedure 5

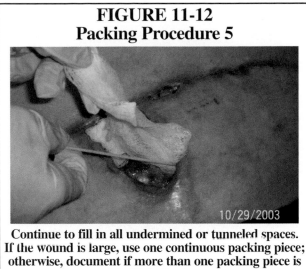

Continue to fill in all undermined or tunneled spaces. If the wound is large, use one continuous packing piece; otherwise, document if more than one packing piece is used to fill in dead space.

Photograph provided by Vivian Sternweiler, MS, RN, CWCN. Reprinted with permission.

FIGURE 11-13
Packing Procedure 6

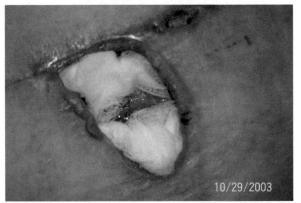

At this point, all undermined or tunneled areas have been packed.

Photograph provided by Vivian Sternweiler, MS, RN, CWCN. Reprinted with permission.

FIGURE 11-14
Packing Procedure 7

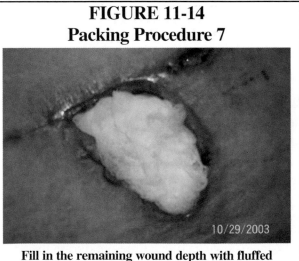

Fill in the remaining wound depth with fluffed open packing material.

Photograph provided by Vivian Sternweiler, MS, RN, CWCN. Reprinted with permission.

FIGURE 11-15
Packing Procedure 8

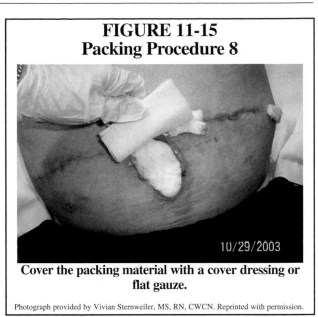

Cover the packing material with a cover dressing or flat gauze.

Photograph provided by Vivian Sternweiler, MS, RN, CWCN. Reprinted with permission.

SECURING THE DRESSING

Keeping the dressing secure is an important aspect of wound care because, if the dressing remains in place, it has a better chance of enhancing the wound healing principles. Securing the dressing depends on whether the dressing is a primary dressing, secondary dressing, adhesive, or nonadhesive. A primary dressing comes in contact with the wound bed and may also be a cover dressing. A secondary dressing is one that is applied over the primary dressing, which comes in contact with the wound bed. Some of the cover dressings are one piece, including the adhesive, and others are simply made of a gauze type material that needs to be secured.

The frequency of dressing changes, type of dressing, and protection of the periwound skin are also factors to consider when choosing a method to secure the dressing. The use of skin preparation along with paper tape or breathable tape may be an acceptable choice. Hydrocolloid strips may be used around the perimeter of the wound to attach the dressing without continued irritation of the skin. Montgomery straps, tubular mesh or netting, support belts, undergarments, and elastic wraps are also options that can be used to secure a dressing, especially one that is changed more often, as well as protect the periwound skin (see Figure 11-16). Specialty tapes such as 3-M's Medipore™ tape or Smith & Nephew's Hypafix® Dressing Retention tape assist in securing the dressing while limiting skin injury with application and removal. These tapes also conform well to different skin surfaces and curves (Bryant, 2000). (See Figures 11-17 & 11-18.)

FIGURE 11-16
Options for Securing a Dressing

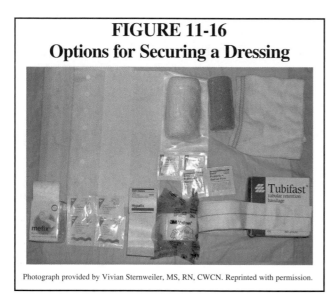

Photograph provided by Vivian Sternweiler, MS, RN, CWCN. Reprinted with permission.

FIGURE 11-17
Securing a Dressing

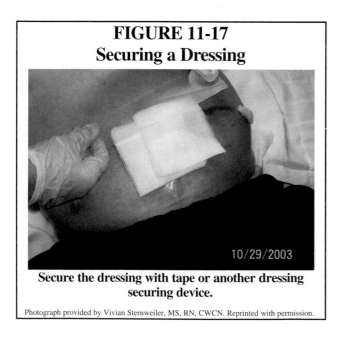

10/29/2003

Secure the dressing with tape or another dressing securing device.

Photograph provided by Vivian Sternweiler, MS, RN, CWCN. Reprinted with permission.

FIGURE 11-18
Labeling a Dressing

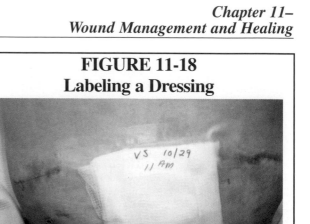

10/29/2003

Always label the dressing change with the date, time, and your initials.

Photograph provided by Vivian Sternweiler, MS, RN, CWCN. Reprinted with permission.

PAIN MANAGEMENT WITH DRESSING CHANGES

One of the goals when changing a wound dressing is to make the procedure as painless as possible for the patient. Some of the more traditional dressing changes, such as wet-to-dry dressing changes, are associated with wound pain because the dressing is allowed to dry out, thereby sticking to the wound bed or necrotic tissue and pulling upon removal of the dressing. Some of the wound bed or necrosis may be removed as well. This act usually is quite painful for the patient. Many times, the clinician, moistens the dressing to decrease the pain associated with wet-to-dry dressings. Doing so, however, renders this type of dressing ineffective.

Krasner and Kane (2001) discuss wound pain and label the pain associated with repeated dressing changes, wound interventions, or turning and positioning as cyclic acute wound pain. Interventions for this type of wound pain include both pharmacological and nonpharmacological options. Topical and systemic analgesia can be used, but nonpharmacological interventions, such as using pain-reducing dressings, having the patient assist in the dressing change, taking a time-out during the dressing change, and choosing a time for the dressing change when the patient is most receptive, all appear to have a benefit in reducing wound pain. Using pressure-relieving devices and utilizing positioning to decrease wound pain during the dressing change also are effective methods.

The advances that have been made to dressings in the wound care setting have improved the amount of pain a patient has with the dressing change. The shift to moist wound healing principles has allowed for improvements in dressings that provide some moisture to the wound base while preventing adhesion of the dressing to the wound bed thereby reducing pain. If the patient still has pain with the dressing change, the etiology of the wound and pain should be reevaluated. Topical or systemic analgesia can be administered but should be agreed upon by the wound care team (Bryant, 2000).

CLEAN VERSUS STERILE TECHNIQUE FOR THE DRESSING CHANGE

The use of clean versus sterile technique for wound care has been an issue of great debate within the wound care community for several years. The answer to this issue has still not been resolved. Barber (2002) reviewed the literature from the last 5 years and found that there is no standard answer for when to use clean versus sterile technique. Nurses were inclined to base the decision on the setting of the client, the client's overall status, and the severity of the wound. Governmental policies on clean versus sterile technique only come from the Agency for Healthcare Research and Quality (AHRQ) and the Centers for Disease Control and Prevention (CDC) and are limited in scope. The AHRQ recommends clean or nonsterile technique when pressure ulcers are managed. The CDC recommends sterile glove use for the first 24 hours postoperatively for incision care. Other than these specific recommendations, standards for clean versus sterile technique are limited.

In 1997, a pilot study by Stotts et al. looked at sterile versus clean technique in postoperative wound care of patients with open surgical wounds. The previous management of open surgical wounds was performed with sterile technique because it had been assumed that this type of wound care was necessary to achieve wound healing and prevent infection. With additional wound care research, findings showed that open surgical wounds healing by secondary intention were colonized with the patient's own normal flora, but these wounds were found to go on to healing with out any difficulty. The study was conducted to see if sterile technique really was necessary with these colonized wounds. The study was conducted with 30 subjects who had undergone abdominal surgery. The subjects were randomly assigned to either clean or sterile dressing changes and all other protocols for the usual treatment of wounds was maintained. The results of the study showed no difference in healing rates between the clean versus sterile dressing change groups. The study did show that clean dressings and techniques were less expensive than the sterile counterpart. A limitation of the study was that the sample size was small; confirming results with a larger study group would be helpful.

In another wound care study, Wise, Hoffman, Grant, & Bostrom (1997) conducted a prospective, descriptive study of staff nurses' choices in using sterile versus nonsterile gloves when providing wound care. The study found that a nurse's choice of glove, whether it was sterile or nonsterile, dictated how the rest of the wound care or dressing change was to be conducted. The choice for clean gloves meant that the remaining wound care would be done with clean technique; if sterile gloves were chosen, the remaining dressing change would be sterile. Even though these findings were present, no clear guidelines have been set on the use of glove type when performing wound care.

Barber (2002) also noted that the terms "clean technique" and "sterile technique" mean different things to different individuals and that health care providers practice both techniques in similar and different situations. There have also been attempts in the wound care community to mesh the two terms together, creating more confusion. Basically, there is no clear and convincing research-based evidence to choose one dressing change method over another. Clinicians must rely on general wound care principles that they have learned, adhere to agency policy with regard to wound care practices, and follow governmental guidelines that are available from the CDC and the AHRQ until more researched-based studies have been performed.

SUMMARY

The act of changing a wound dressing may appear to be a simple task, but several principles must be maintained in order to obtain the best outcome for wound repair and patient comfort. It is important that the clinician be well versed on the type of wound products that are being used for the dressing change, because specific categories of wound care products are designed to be applied and removed in a specific fashion in order to facilitate wound healing, protect the periwound skin, and provide the patient with as little discomfort as possible. Infection control measures must always be kept in mind in every clinical setting to control bacteria management and provide a hygienic environment. Universal precautions are the gold standard to maintain. The use of clean versus sterile technique in the dressing change continues to be quite controversial, and no evidence-based research has proven one method better than the other. The clinician needs to follow agency policy in this area.

CHAPTER 11
Questions 91-95

91. An effective method of removing a dressing to limit injury to the client's skin is to

    a. remove the dressing in the opposite direction that hair is growing.

    b. remove the dressing in the same direction that hair is growing.

    c. cut all adhesive off dressings before removing them.

    d. remove the dressing in one, quick jerk to limit the time the patient will be in pain.

92. An appropriate method of packing a wound is to

    a. leave a tail of the packing exposed when tunneling or undermining are present.

    b. pack the dead space in the wound loosely by only 1/3 to allow for air to get into the wound bed.

    c. pack the dead space in the wound very tightly.

    d. avoid packing tunnels and undermining so that drainage can escape into the main wound.

93. What option is a poor choice to use to secure a dressing when there is injury to the surrounding skin?

    a. The use of Montgomery straps

    b. The use of hydrocolloid strips to apply the dressing tape to

    c. The use of surgical netting

    d. Continued use of the current taping system even though it may be causing irritation

94. An option to decrease pain with the dressing change is to

    a. use wet-to-dry dressing changes.

    b. increase the frequency of dressing change.

    c. have the client participate in the dressing change.

    d. hurry up and remove the dressing as fast as possible.

95. Current literature on clean versus sterile technique states that

    a. sterile supplies must be used with pressure ulcers.

    b. sterile supplies must be used with surgical wounds.

    c. clean supplies must be used with surgical wounds.

    d. there are no specific guidelines on when to use sterile versus clean technique.

CHAPTER 12

ADJUNCTIVE WOUND CARE THERAPIES

CHAPTER OBJECTIVE

Upon completion of this chapter, the reader will be able to discuss adjunctive therapies that are available for use in the management of wounds and how these therapies can enhance wound resolution.

LEARNING OBJECTIVES

Upon completion of the chapter, the reader will be able to

1. name one growth factor that is used in the treatment of neuropathic ulcers.

2. identify three types of wounds for which vacuum-assisted wound closure therapy can be used.

3. state two names of bioengineered skin that can be used as a permanent skin covering for the treatment of full-thickness wounds.

INTRODUCTION

The management of wounds during the last several years has been focused on moist wound healing and the products or practices that support this approach. This basic tenet is still in force as a fundamental aspect of wound management, yet the science of wound healing has progressed to include more frequent use of adjunctive therapies. In the past, these therapies were mainly used for the recalcitrant wound that appeared stagnant. The latest research on many of these adjunctive therapies shows that they can be beneficial to wound healing with routine use. Adjunctive therapies, such as hyperbaric oxygen, vacuum-assisted wound closure, growth factors, electrical stimulation, and bioengineered skin, are being used more frequently to complete the goals of wound management and healing. The future of these therapies appears very promising, as newer applications are being studied and approved for various types of wound management.

HYPERBARIC OXYGEN

Hyperbaric oxygen (HBO) is 100% oxygen that is delivered under pressure greater than 1 atmosphere to the patient. This type of oxygen is delivered in a systemic and intermittent way to enhance the amount of oxygen in the tissues and, therefore, improve wound healing. HBO was originally used for decompression sickness in deep-sea divers and for carbon monoxide poisoning but has been used in the last several years for conditions in which the underlying pathophysiology is tissue hypoxia. Disease states, such as peripheral vascular disease, diabetes, irradiation, crush injury, and compromised skin flaps and grafts, all contribute to the formation of chronic wounds and yield a hypoxic state.

In HBO, the patient is placed into a chamber that may hold a single patient or several patients. The patient then breathes in oxygen. The atmospheric pressure gradually rises, causing the oxygen to dissolve in the plasma at higher concentrations than would normally be seen at sea level. The hemoglobin in the blood stream becomes supersaturated with oxygen and is able to deliver a greater supply of oxygen to the tissues (Bryant, 2000; Maklebust & Sieggreen, 2001).

The immune system, wound healing, and vascular tone are all affected by the levels of oxygen in the tissues. Intermittent HBO treatments help to stimulate the oxidative functions of wound healing, allowing greater availability of oxygen to the vital cells, such as fibroblasts, leukocytes, and endothelial cells. Increasing the oxygen level assists with the conditions that lead to hypoxia. Wound healing is thought to be optimal when periods of oxygenation are alternated with periods of relative hypoxia.

Systemic HBO therapy is used in the management of wounds. Topical HBO therapy is not recommended, because treatment with topical oxygen does not increase the tissue oxygen tension beyond the superficial dermis, so the needed effect of the oxygen does not occur. The clinician must also remember that a wound that is poorly perfused due to arterial insufficiency or other factors must have those contributing factors addressed first in order to restore optimal blood flow and potential for healing. HBO therapy does not get to the tissues if poor vascular flow is present. The use of HBO requires specialized facilities and personnel. HBO therapy also has its risks and contraindications. Clinicians who are considering placing a patient on HBO therapy need to discuss the therapy with an HBO specialist (Maklebust & Sieggreen, 2001; Milne, Corbett, & Dubuc, 2003).

GROWTH FACTORS

Growth factors are polypeptide molecules that influence growth, differentiation, and metabolism of cells while the wound healing process is in progress. Growth factors are secreted by many types of cells involved in wound healing, such as fibroblasts, platelets, inflammatory cells, and epithelial cells. They assist in promoting new granulation tissue and the process of epithelialization to cover the wound base. Growth factors interact with cells at the local level to enhance the rate of wound repair in the chronic wound. These molecules work within a network of factors that interact to produce the desired effect. Different growth factors target different cells, yet a single growth factor may target more than one cell.

An example of a topically applied growth factor that is used in wound management is rh-PDGF-BB (becaplermin). The trade name of this growth factor is Regranex® and it is distributed by Johnson & Johnson Wound Management Worldwide. A few key concepts to note with Regranex® include: a) as of this writing, the product has only been approved by the FDA for use in diabetic neuropathic ulcers; b) the product needs to remain refrigerated for stability; c) the product needs to be used in wounds that are free from necrosis in order for the growth factor to be effective; d) the recommended dressing change frequency is every 12 hours, during which the Regranex® dressing is placed on the wound for the first 12 hours and then the dressing is changed to a normal saline dressing for the next 12 hours; e) the product is placed on the wound at about the thickness of a dime; and f) the shelf life is relatively short so the expiration date should be monitored. The research on using growth factors in wound healing is increasing as more information becomes known about the mechanisms of action and the possible benefits (Bryant, 2000; Maklebust & Sieggreen, 2001).

ULTRASOUND

Ultrasound therapy for wound management is a modality that is most often used by the discipline of physical therapy. In ultrasound therapy, high-frequency sound waves are generated by the oscillation of a crystal transducer, either in a continuous mode or in a pulsed interrupted mode, to affect wound healing. The therapeutic effect of ultrasound is thought to occur when sound waves cross the cell wall, causing a change in the diffusion rate and cell membrane permeability, which is thought to affect the wound healing rate. In a clinical study, ultrasound therapy appeared to accelerate the rate of the inflammatory phase of wound healing. However, not many studies have been conducted on the use of ultrasound therapy with wound healing; more research is needed on this therapy (Maklebust & Sieggreen, 2001).

VACUUM-ASSISTED WOUND CLOSURE

Vacuum-assisted wound closure, or negative-pressure wound therapy, is used to assist and accelerate wound closure. This therapy is also known as VAC® (KCI, San Antonio, Texas) therapy. This type of adjunctive therapy is used to reduce the bacterial burden in the wound; decrease tissue edema by evacuation of wound fluid, which improves blood flow to the area; stimulate granulation tissue formation; and assist in a more uniform closure of wounds. An open-cell foam sponge dressing is placed inside the wound and then the foam is sealed with a transparent, adhesive dressing. A plastic tube is connected from the sponge to a computerized pump. The pump provides negative pressure to the foam dressing, creating the vacuum. The pump can be programmed to provide either continuous or intermittent suction as well as the desired amount of negative pressure.

Vacuum-assisted wound closure is indicated for pressure ulcers, vascular ulcers, acute wounds, skin flaps and grafts, dehisced wounds, diabetic ulcers, and chronic wounds from a variety of etiologies. The device may be used on infected wounds that are concurrently being treated with antibiotics as well as treated osteomyelitis. Contraindications of negative-pressure wound therapy include wounds with necrotic tissue, malignant wounds, untreated osteomyelitis, and wounds with exposed arteries and veins. Precautions must be instituted for individuals who are on anticoagulant therapy, have a bleeding disorder, or have fistulas to an organ.

The vacuum-assisted wound closure device should be off for no more than 2 hours out of 24. The VAC dressing is changed every 12 hours for active infection or every 48 hours for general care. In such settings as home health or skilled facilities, the VAC dressing is changed three times per week, on Monday, Wednesday, and Friday, with the dressing being left in place for the weekend. The standard amount of negative pressure used in many wounds is 125 mm Hg, although this can be adjusted depending on the type of wound. Vascular ulcers may require less negative pressure and the pressure may need to be lowered to 75 mm Hg. Split thickness skin grafts are another instance in which the pressure may need to be lowered to a range of 15 to 100 mm Hg. Negative-pressure therapy for skin grafts is usually done on a continuous basis for approximately 5 days. The foam dressing is not changed during this 5-day duration unless a problem is present (Bryant, 2000; Hess, 2002).

BIOENGINEERED SKIN

The use of bioengineered skin is becoming more of a standard management technique in the treatment of wounds. Bioengineered skin, or a skin substitute, can be used as either a temporary or permanent covering to replace skin that has been lost or damaged after trauma or burns or with chronic wounds. Skin substitutes are manufactured in various ways and can be placed directly in or over the wound. Some bioengineered skin substitutes are used for partial-thickness wounds and other skin substitutes are used for full-thickness wounds.

The most common skin substitutes used in partial-thickness burns are TransCyte™ and Biobrane.® TransCyte is a temporary skin substitute manufactured from human fibroblasts that helps to provide a temporary epidermis. Biobrane is manufactured as a biosynthetic wound dressing made of a silicone film with a nylon fabric partially enmeshed into the film. These temporary skin substitutes are used to decrease pain, improve healing rate, and decrease the number of dressing changes required. These benefits help to improve the quality of life that the burn patient endures during the healing phase.

Bioengineered skin substitutes that are used on full-thickness wounds to provide a permanent dermal covering include Integra,® AlloDerm,® Apligraf,® and Dermagraft.® Integra and AlloDerm are approved for use on full-thickness burns. Dermagraft and Apligraf are approved for use on neuropathic ulcers and venous ulcers, but trials are ongoing with uses for other chronic wounds, such as traumatic wounds and arterial ulcers. These skin substitutes have growth factors, cytokines, and matrix proteins that all promote improved healing and resolution of wounds.

AlloDerm is a processed human cadaver allograft that is immunologically inert. After AlloDerm is applied, most often for surgically excised wounds, an ultrathin split-thickness skin graft from the patient is applied during the same operation. This autograft allows for final closure of the wound. Integra is produced as a bilayered dermal regeneration template, in which the dermal layer is manufactured of bovine collagen. This dermal replacement layer functions as a matrix for the infiltration of macrophages, lymphocytes, fibroblasts, and capillaries. The outer layer that is made of silicone serves as the temporary epidermal covering until an autograft is placed on top. It takes approximately 14–21 days for the incorporation of the patient's own cells to infiltrate into the Integra matrix, creating a neodermis that will then accept the patient's autograft. Integra is often used for the postexcisional treatment of deep partial-thickness or full-thickness burns when an autograft is not available in sufficient amounts.

Apligraf is considered an allogenic, cultured skin equivalent that has both an epidermal and dermal layer. The use of bioengineered human fibroblasts assists in the formation of the dermal layer. The epidermal layer comes from bioengineered keratinocytes. Apligraf does not have macrophages, lymphocytes, Langerhan's cells, melanocytes, or blood vessels in its matrix. The human fibroblasts and keratinocytes are obtained from neonatal foreskin, from which the cells are removed during the manufacturing process. Dermagraft is also a cultured skin equivalent in which human dermal fibroblasts are isolated from the foreskin of a newborn after circumcision. The fibroblasts are separated from the tissue and seeded onto a bioabsorbable scaffold of vicryl mesh. Approximately 2 weeks after the fibroblasts have been seeded, a living dermal substitute has been formed that supports the migration and proliferation of an epidermis (Bryant, 2000; Krasner & Kane, 2001; Milne, Corbett, & Dubuc, 2003).

ELECTRICAL STIMULATION

Electrical stimulation is a wound healing modality that is usually performed by a physical therapist. Research has found that the human body resembles a battery. Electrical current can flow from one skin area to another if the circuit is complete. This process is termed current of injury. The outer portion of the skin is electronegative with regard to the deeper tissues, which are positively charged, and to wound tissues, which are positively charged. Electrical stimulation mimics the natural currents of energy in the body trying to correct the damage to the human skin bioelectric process. The application of high-voltage pulsed direct electrical current, current to the wound causes the release of the body's natural endorphins. This application of electric current to the wound leaves a net-charge depending on what type of electrode was used. The net-charge, which is either positive or negative in the wound, has been shown to stimulate wound healing.

High-voltage pulsed current helps with wound healing by stimulating angiogenesis and epithelial migration. Several protocols are available to the clinician for electrical stimulation. Regimens of therapy vary depending on the phase of healing and area of wound involvement. Electrical stimulation is indicated when wounds have not responded to other wound treatment, angiogenesis is the goal, pain control is warranted, and range of motion of the wounded area is increased. Contraindications for electrical stimulation include malignancy, electrical implant or pacemaker, use over a pregnant uterus, use over metal ions, active osteomyelitis, and use over the upper chest and anterior neck (because of the presence of vital organs and reflex centers). Because there are many facets to electrical stimulation, the clinician needs to seek information from qualified therapists when considering this therapy.

RADIANT HEAT THERAPY

Radiant heat therapy is based on the premise that most wounds are hypothermic, averaging 5.6° F cooler that the core body temperature, and if wounds are warmed up to the core temperature, healing is accelerated. General research on wound healing has shown that hypothermia causes vasoconstriction, lowers collagen deposition in the wound base, and depresses neutrophil activity, which all delay wound healing. Radiant heat therapy is one method of warming the wound to prevent the detrimental effects of hypothermia. At the time of this printing, only one form of radiant heat therapy is available, Warm-Up Wound Therapy® by Augustine Medical, Inc. Warm-Up Wound Therapy is a system that warms the wound toward normothermia. The warming device is designed to improve blood flow to the wound, increasing subcutaneous oxygen tension and increasing the delivery of growth factors to the wound base. The Warm-Up system maintains appropriate levels of temperature and moisture in the wound and around the wound margins to promote a beneficial environment for healing.

The Warm-Up Wound Therapy system consists of a temperature control unit, an AC adapter, asterile wound cover, and a warming card. The sterile wound cover is a noncontact cover that is placed over the wound and consists of a water-resistant thin shell with an adhesive border that sticks to the intact skin around the wound. The cover has a clear window for wound observation, and a pocket within the clear window holds the warming card over the wound. The foam frame helps to absorb exudate and protect the wound from trauma and contamination. The warming card is placed into the window frame for 1 hour three times per day to achieve the recommended amount of radiant therapy.

Indications for radiant heat therapy include venous, arterial, pressure, and neuropathic ulcers. Wounds that are infected may be treated with the therapy as long as concurrent antibiotic therapy is instituted. This therapy is contraindicated for third-degree burns (Hess, 2002).

SUMMARY

The art and science of wound management combine general principles of wound healing that include looking at the etiology of the wound, the host factors that affect wound healing, both internal and external, and the options available to treat the wound. Wound treatment always involves correction of the etiology, improvement of the host factors for healing, and then evaluation of the most appropriate topical treatment. It is still prudent to follow the principles of moist wound healing, which provide the optimal environment for healing. Numerous products are available to obtain this goal. However, the research on adjunctive therapies, such as hyperbaric oxygen, growth factors, vacuum-assisted wound closure, ultrasound, electrical stimulation, and bioengineered tissues, shows excellent results, with enhanced wound healing and closure.

Therefore, these therapies should not be only on the recalcitrant wound. These therapies should be thought of as viable options early on in the wound treatment plan because the goals of wound healing are to close the wound, if possible, and return the patient to the most function level possible.

CHAPTER 12
Questions 96-98

96. The independent growth factor that has been approved for use in neuropathic ulcers is

    a. hydrogel.
    b. rh-PDGF-BB.
    c. HBO.
    d. VEGF.

97. Vacuum-assisted wound closure can be used on

    a. vascular ulcers, neoplastic lesions, and fistulas.
    b. pressure ulcers, neoplastic lesions, and fistulas.
    c. neuropathic ulcers, pressure ulcers, and skin flaps.
    d. pressure ulcers, untreated osteomyelitis, and vascular ulcers.

98. Types of bioengineered skin that can be used as permanent skin coverings include

    a. HBO and Integra.
    b. Apligraf and Dermagraft.
    c. Integra and TransCyte.
    d. TransCyte and Biobrane.

CHAPTER 13

REIMBURSEMENT PRACTICES

CHAPTER OBJECTIVE

Upon completion of the chapter, the reader will be able to identify some of the payor sources available for reimbursement of wound care services and steps that can be taken to ensure successful reimbursement.

LEARNING OBJECTIVES

After completion of the chapter, the reader will be able to

1. distinguish between Medicare, Medicaid/ MediCal, and Health Maintenance Organization (HMO) reimbursement.

2. state two areas of cost containment for wound management.

INTRODUCTION

Reimbursement issues are always an important component of any health care service. The Balanced Budget Act of 1997 caused significant changes in health care delivery, especially in the home health and skilled nursing facility settings. In the past, payment for wound care products and services varied depending on whether the patient had primary coverage from Medicare, Medicaid/MediCal, or an HMO-type plan. Depending on the patient's setting, the dressings or products could be billed separately or lumped together as a per diem cost

with adjustments made to that cost on a yearly basis. The Balanced Budget Act decreased the reimbursement per episode of illness from Medicare that any agency or facility will be paid to treat its members. These changes made it especially important for health care clinicians to understand the most appropriate and cost-effective methods for treating patients with acute or chronic wounds. The health care industry has since settled into this new payment system and has adapted itself in order to continue to provide appropriate health care services. This chapter reviews the general practices of reimbursement payors including Medicare, MediCal, and health maintenance organizations (HMOs). The final portion of this chapter provides some general information that can be used to make the reimbursement process more successful. This chapter does not discuss billing or reimbursement practices in detail because they vary across the country.

REIMBURSEMENT PAYOR MIX

The area of the United States in which the clinician practices affects the major payor mix. Medicare and Medicaid/MediCal have been the primary payors over the last several years for health care expenses, especially in the home health arena. This has, however, changed in certain parts of the country as managed care has grown in its acceptance. This chapter discusses Medicare in detail but starts off with Medicaid/MediCal and managed care systems.

MEDICAID/MEDICAL

The Medicaid/MediCal programs and their equivalents are programs of medical assistance that have joint funding by the states and the federal government. They are designed for impoverished individuals who are aged, blind, disabled, or members of families with dependent children. The programs are administered by the state under the direction of federal guidelines. Each state's program can vary widely within the main framework of the federal guidelines. Because each state's program varies, the reimbursement for wound care products and services also varies. It is important to check with the payor on their policies concerning coverage for wound care. Some products or services require a Treatment Authorization Request (TAR) or some other type of documentation to be filled out. It is important to inquire about required documentation, reimbursement mechanisms, and payment levels prior to initiating services.

MANAGED CARE/HMO

The managed care programs, also known as HMOs, offer a variety of options for providing services, either to employers or individuals, as well as to seniors in place of their Medicare benefits. Senior managed care plans follow Medicare guidelines for many of their services yet can institute their own policies with regard to certain services or covered items. HMOs also have a variety of options when it comes to covered items such as supplies. Many times, supplies such as wound care products or services are built into a per diem rate that the managed care plan offers. The individual may be required to pay for supplies or to pay for some portion of the supplies. In this regard, once again, it is important to inquire about how wound care supplies

are obtained, what type of reimbursement is available, and what documentation may be necessary for reimbursement.

MEDICARE

The Medicare plan is the largest national payor for supplies and services in the health care arena, especially in the home health setting. Depending on the payor mix in a particular geographic area, Medicare remains an important force in overall reimbursement. The fact that Medicare plays such a large role in reimbursement is the reason that the Balanced Budget Act of 1997 created such interest and controversy. Medicare traditionally has been divided into two benefits: Part A and Part B.

Part A: Institutional insurance coverage that includes benefits for hospital, skilled nursing facility, home health care, and hospice services.

Part B: Supplemental insurance coverage that provides benefits for physician's services, outpatient services, diagnostic procedures, medical supplies, prosthetic devices, and durable medical equipment.

Medicare Part A

Wound care supplies reimbursed under Part A for the home health setting and the skilled setting are distributed under the prospective payment system, or PPS. For a home health agency, reimbursement is a set amount to cover a 60-day period of patient care that should cover the agency's expenses. The completion of the Outcome Assessment and Information Set (OASIS) form determines the reimbursement amount. The OASIS data place the patient at an acuity level. All patient expenses, including the skilled nursing visit, wound care supplies, and other supplies, are provided by the home health agency while home health care is being delivered. The financial success of a home health agency is impacted by the accuracy of OASIS data.

The management of wound care supplies in a

skilled nursing facility for Medicare Part A is also provided under the PPS system. A resident of a skilled nursing facility is assessed on admission and on days 5, 14, 30, 60, and 90. For each of these assessments, the resident is grouped into a category that will provide a reimbursement rate to the facility. This reimbursement rate covers all services and supplies that the facility needs to provide to the resident. It is imperative that a Resident Assessment Instrument (RAI) form be filled out appropriately at each assessment interval in order for the facility to receive adequate reimbursement to cover such items as wound care supplies (Milne, Corbett, & Dubuc, 2003).

Medicare Part B

Medicare Part B may be used to bill for wound care supplies in the home health setting and in a skilled nursing facility. Under Medicare Part B, wound care supplies can be billed when home health care is no longer being provided or the patient at the skilled nursing facility is considered to be on a custodial status. A medical supply dealer who furnishes the supplies to the beneficiary bills Medicare. Medicare then directs the payment to the medical supply dealer for the 80% assigned claim and notifies the beneficiary of the 20% copayment due. The difference between reimbursement for supplies under Part A and Part B is that Part B requires the following conditions:

- The beneficiary assumes a portion of the cost of the medical supplies.

- The only covered supplies include "primary and secondary surgical dressings."

A thorough definition of primary and secondary dressings can be found in the Medicare Carriers Manual, which has the surgical dressing policy. This policy is very specific as to the types of dressings covered, frequency of dressing changes, and the types of wounds for which these dressings are most effective. Special codes that coincide with each dressing type must be utilized when billing occurs. The claims for surgical dressings provided

to Medicare patients are sent to the regional insurance carriers responsible for claims processing in the state where the beneficiary has a permanent residence. These carriers are called Durable Medical Equipment Regional Carriers, or DMERCs. There are four DMERCs in the country (see Figure 13-1).

Information on reimbursement through the DMERC carriers can be obtained online through several web sites by searching for durable medical equipment regional carriers. If a dressing does not meet the criteria outlined by the surgical dressing policy, the beneficiary is responsible for 100% of the cost (Hess, 2002).

ADDITIONAL STEPS FOR REIMBURSEMENT SUCCESS

As stated above, most payors have instituted some form of PPS that forces health care providers to manage skin and wound care very closely. Today's wound management needs to be tied to cost-effective, quality outcomes that focus on patient satisfaction and maintain the quality assurance that the payors expect. To be successful in this environment takes diligence to keep up with the changes in wound management and reimbursement. Health care providers need to carefully review contracts with all payors to determine coverage criteria, coding, and payment reimbursement rates for procedures, services, and products that are used in patient care. It is also important for the provider to understand how the patient will obtain supplies if orders are written because this can become a road block for follow through on wound management. There are times when the health care provider may have to prescribe a less than optimal plan of treatment due to financial constraints. Complete data should be kept on these instances so that payors can review the outcomes of these cases (Hess, 2002).

FIGURE 13-1:
DURABLE MEDICAL EQUIPMENT REGIONAL CARRIERS

Region	Carrier	States/Regions Covered
Region A	Healthnow NY, Inc. DMERC A P. O. Box 6800 Wilkes-Barre, PA 18773-6800 866-419-9458	Connecticut, Delaware, Maine, Massachusetts, New Hampshire, New Jersey, New York, Pennsylvania, Rhode Island, Vermont
Region B	AdminaStar Federal, Inc. DMERC Region B Service Office P. O. Box 7027 Indianapolis, IN 46207 877-299-7900	District of Columbia, Illinois, Indiana, Maryland, Michigan, Minnesota, Ohio, Virginia, West Virginia, Wisconsin
Region C	Palmetto Government Benefits Administrators Medicare DMERC Operators P. O. Box 100141 Columbia, SC 29292-3141 866-238-9650	Alabama, Arkansas, Colorado, Florida, Georgia, Kentucky, Louisiana, Mississippi, New Mexico, North Carolina, Oklahoma, Puerto Rico, South Carolina, Tennessee, Texas, Virgin Islands
Region D	Medicare DMERC Region D P. O. Box 690 Nashville, TN 37202 877-320-0390	Alaska, Arizona, California, Guam, Hawaii, Idaho, Iowa, Kansas, Missouri, Montana, Nebraska, Nevada, North Dakota, Oregon, South Dakota, Utah, Washington, Wyoming

Providers can institute the following steps to assist in achieving clinical and financial reimbursement goals

- Have written policies and procedures that apply to the management of skin and wound care.

- Obtain cost controls and reductions with volume purchases and try to standardize the products.

- Obtain services of wound and skin care specialists to assist in developing a wound management program.

- Develop wound care maps or pathways that are research-based to guide wound and skin management.

- Develop a wound and skin care formulary that is effective, efficient, and readily available.

- Allow technology to work for the wound program. Utilize products, services that have been tested to decrease the number of professional visits, total cost of care, and time to heal.

- Institute a delivery system that prevents inventory buildup or a delay in obtaining supplies.

- Have a system in place to manage medical waste.

- Have a photo documentation system in place.

- Make a list of all ICD-9, CPT, HCPCS, Pass-through, and New Technology codes that assist in correct identification of medical diagnosis, evaluation, treatments, services, and products utilized in the management of wound care.

- Develop a way to track wound management outcomes.

- Keep excellent wound assessment and documentation data to track wound outcomes.

- Develop a program of patient and family education on wound management that includes wound healing modalities and supplies.

- Establish a method of wound documentation that facilitates coordination and collaboration with physicians as well as other disciplines involved in the management wound and skin care.

- Institute timely referrals to other levels of care or resources. (Hess, 2002)

SUMMARY

The management of wound care involves many facets. Not only do clinicians need a sound knowledge base on the principles of wound healing but also on the cost-effective management of the supplies and services that are rendered in that care. The payors in the health care arena today have access to a large amount of research and information that helps guide them in their decisions to control costs while obtaining the most appropriate care for their beneficiaries. As health care providers, clinicians and agency personnel are required to keep abreast of the changes in treatment for wound care as well as the changes in reimbursement, not only from the federal and state governments but also from private payors, managed care plans, and combined payors as well. Even though reimbursement practices have changed over the last few years, it is possible to provide cost-effective, appropriate wound and skin care to patients and still remain financially sound. Achieving clinical and financial goals is possible with excellent planning for wound and skin care delivery and meticulous documentation of wound care outcomes.

EXAM QUESTIONS

CHAPTER 13
Questions 99-100

99. The type of payor that tends to follow Medicare guidelines for reimbursement of wound care products but still has the ability to adjust their own policies with regard to certain services is

    a. Medicaid.
    b. Medicare.
    c. health maintenance organizations.
    d. private pay plans.

100. What measure can be taken by the health care provider to provide cost-effective wound care?

    a. Purchase supplies in small amounts.
    b. Develop wound care maps to assist with wound management.
    c. Do not institute new technology in wound care because it has not been tested.
    d. Wait to obtain any referrals or consults for wound assistance until numerous trials of topical products have failed.

This concludes the final examination.

RESOURCES

Agency for Health Care Policy and Research
(AHCPR) Clinical Practice Guidelines
www.ahrq.org

National Pressure Ulcer Advisory Panel
www.npuap.org

Wound, Ostomy, and Continence Nurses Society
(WOCN)
www.wocn.org

A comprehensive list of products available
for wound care, including companies,
order numbers, and contacts
www.woundsource.com

GLOSSARY

abscess: Localized collection of pus in any part of the body as a result of acute or chronic localized infection.

acute wound: Wound that is created traumatically or surgically, usually requires limited local wound care, and usually follows the healing trajectory.

aerobe: Microorganism that lives and grows in the presence of free oxygen.

anaerobe: Microorganism that lives and grows in the absence of free oxygen.

angiogenesis: Development of new blood vessels.

ankle-brachial index (ABI): Noninvasive vascular assessment test to determine vascular (arterial) flow. The test is performed with the use of a Doppler ultrasound to obtain the ankle systolic pressure and the brachial systolic pressure, which result in a ratio that is an indicator of arterial flow.

antibacterial: Agent that inhibits the growth of bacteria.

antimicrobial: Agent that is destructive to microorganisms.

antiseptic (topical): Product with antimicrobial activity designed for use on skin or other superficial tissues; may damage cells.

arterial ulcer: Ulcer caused by ischemia; related to the presence of arterial occlusive disease.

autolysis: Disintegration or liquefaction of tissue or cells by the body's own mechanisms (leukocytes or enzymes).

avascular: Tissues without blood or lymphatic vessels.

bacteremia: Presence of viable bacteria in the circulating blood.

bactericidal: Agent that destroys bacteria.

bacteriostatic: Agent that is capable of inhibiting the growth or multiplication of bacteria.

bioengineered skin: Skin substitute that is manufactured from human fibroblasts and keratinocytes and used as either a temporary or permanent covering to replace skin that has been lost or damaged.

body substance isolation (BSI): System of infection control procedures routinely used with all patients to prevent cross-contamination of pathogens. The system emphasizes the use of barrier precautions to isolate potentially infectious body substances.

bottoming out: Expression used to describe inadequate support from a mattress overlay or seat cushion as determined by a "hand check." To perform a hand check, the nurse places an outstretched hand palm up under the overlay or cushion below the pressure ulcer or the part of the body at risk for a pressure ulcer. If the nurse feels less than an inch of support material, the patient has "bottomed out" and the support surface is therefore inadequate.

calor: Heat: one of the four classic signs of inflammation.

cell migration: Movement of cells in the repair process.

cellulitis: Inflammation of cellular or connective tissue characterized by redness, swelling, and tenderness; signifies a spreading infectious process.

Charcot's disease: Rapidly progressive and destructive bone and joint disease that may be self-limiting; also called diabetic neuropathic arthropathy.

clean: Containing no foreign material or debris.

clean dressing: Dressing that is not sterile but is free from environmental contaminants, such as water damage, dust, pest and rodent contaminants, and gross soiling.

clean wound: Wound that is free from purulent drainage, devitalized tissue, and dirt.

collagen: Main supportive protein of skin, tendon, bone, cartilage, and connective tissue.

colonized: Presence of bacteria on the surface or in the tissue of a wound without indications of infection (purulent exudate, foul odor, or surrounding inflammation).

contaminated: Wound containing bacteria, other microorganisms, or other foreign material. Wounds with bacterial counts of 100,000 organisms per gram of tissue or less are generally considered contaminated; those with higher counts are generally considered infected.

Dakin's solution: Buffered sodium hypochlorite; a bactericidal wound irrigant.

dead space: Cavity remaining in a wound.

debridement: Removal of devitalized tissue and foreign matter from the wound. Four types include

autolytic: Use of synthetic dressings to cover a wound and allow eschar or nonviable tissue to self-digest by the action of enzymes present in wound fluids.

enzymatic (chemical): Topical application of proteolytic substances (enzymes) to break down devitalized tissue.

mechanical: Removal of foreign material and devitalized or contaminated tissue from a wound by physical forces rather than by chemical or autolytic forces.

sharp: Removal of foreign material or devitalized tissue by use of a sharp instrument, such as a scalpel or laser; fastest form of debridement.

debris: Remains of broken down or damaged cells or tissue.

decubitus ulcer: Misnomer for a pressure ulcer.

dehiscence: Separation of the layers of a surgical wound.

delay of flaps: Development and transfer of a flap to a recipient site in more than one step to ensure its vascular supply.

denuded: Loss of the epidermis.

desiccation: Process of drying up.

devitalized tissue: Necrotic (dead) tissue.

direct closure: Direct primary closure with sutures; stretches the skin and creates tension that frequently leads to dehiscence and therefore is seldom used except for small, superficial ulcers.

donor site: Site of the body from which a split-thickness skin graft has been taken or harvested.

eccrine glands: Sweat glands.

edema: Presence of abnormally large amounts of fluid in the interstitial space.

elastin: Protein that can be prepared from various connective tissues.

electrical stimulation: Use of an electrical current to transfer energy to a wound to facilitate healing; type of electricity that is transferred is controlled by the electrical source.

enzymes: Biochemical substances that are capable of breaking down necrotic tissue.

epithelialization: Regeneration of the epidermis across the wound surface.

erythema: Redness of the skin surface produced by vasodilation. Two types include

> **blanchable erythema:** Reddened area that temporarily turns white or pale when fingertip pressure is applied; over a pressure site, it is usually due to the normal reactive hyperemic response.

> **nonblanchable erythema:** Redness that persists when fingertip pressure is applied.

eschar: Thick, necrotic, devitalized tissue.

excoriation: Area of open linear scratches on the skin.

exudate: Accumulation of fluid in a wound; may contain serum, cellular debris, bacteria, and leukocytes.

fascia: Sheet or band of fibrous tissue that lies deep below the skin or encloses muscles and various organs of the body.

fibroblast: Any cell from which connective tissue is developed.

fibroplasia: Development of fibrous tissue in wound healing.

fibrosis: Irreversible hardening of normally soft tissue that is associated with lymphedema and also seen in venous insufficiency (termed "woody leg syndrome").

filiariasis: Disorder associated with secondary lymphedema in which the patient is infected with a larvae that is transmitted to humans from the bite of a mosquito.

fluctuance: Wave-like motion indicative of the presence of fluid; used to describe the appearance of tissue under viable or nonviable skin.

free flap: Procedure involving a muscle-type flap in which the vein and artery are disconnected at the donor site and reconnected to the vessels at the recipient site with the aid of a microscope.

friction: Mechanical force exerted when skin is dragged across a coarse surface such as bed linens.

full thickness: Tissue destruction extending through the dermis to involve the subcutaneous layer and possibly muscle or bone.

gaiter area: Medial aspect of the lower leg and ankle and the area superior to the medial malleolus.

granulation tissue: Pink to beefy red, moist tissue that contains new blood vessels, collagen, fibroblasts, and inflammatory cells in a full-thickness wound.

growth factors: Proteins that affect the proliferation, movement, maturation, and biosynthetic activity of cells.

Hansen's disease: a chronic granulomatous infection caused by *Mycobacterium Leprae* which affects parts of the body particularly skin and nerves; also called leprosy.

healing: Dynamic process that can be monitored and measured in which anatomical and functional integrity is restored. For wounds of the skin, it involves repair of the dermis (granulation tissue formation) and epidermis (epithelialization). Healed wounds represent a spectrum of repair from tissue regeneration to temporary return of anatomical continuity to sustained functional and anatomical result.

healing ridge: Accumulation of collagen that, by days 5–9 after surgery, extends approximately 1 cm on either side of the surgical incision indicating wound progression.

hemosiderin: Iron-containing pigment derived from hemoglobin that's caused by the breakdown of red blood cells.

histologically: Referring to the tissues.

hydrophilic: Substance that attracts moisture.

hydrophobic: Substance that repels moisture.

hydrotherapy: Use of whirlpool or submersion in water for wound cleansing.

hyperbaric oxygen: Oxygen at greater than atmospheric pressure that can be applied either to the whole patient inside a pressurized chamber or to individualized limbs via smaller pressurized chambers.

hyperemia: Presence of excess blood in the vessels; engorgement.

hypergranulation tissue: Increased thickness in the granular layer of the epidermis; sometimes called hypertrophic tissue.

incidence: Rate at which new cases of a condition occur during a specific time period.

induration: Process of becoming extremely hard or firm.

indurosis: Term used to refer to firm tissue that should be soft; is reversible and is associated with lymphedema.

infection: Overgrowth of microorganisms capable of tissue destruction and invasion that is accompanied by local or systemic signs and symptoms.

inflammation: Defensive reaction to tissue injury; involves increased blood flow and capillary permeability, and facilitates physiologic cleanup of a wound. It is accompanied by increased heat, redness, swelling and pain in the affected area.

ischemia: Deficiency of blood supply to a tissue; often leads to tissue necrosis.

lesion: Broad term used to refer to wounds or sores.

lymphedema: Swelling that arises when protein-rich fluid collects in the tissues as a direct result of some type of compromise of the lymphatic system; includes plasma proteins, which further attract water and increases the swelling or edema in the interstitial spaces.

keratinocytes: Cells in the epidermis that produce keratin, a tough protein substance found in hair, nails, and skin.

leukocyte: Another name for a neutrophil, or white blood cell.

maceration: Process of softening by wetting or soaking. The degenerative changes and disintegration of skin when it has been kept too moist.

macrophages: Cells that have the ability to destroy bacteria and devitalize tissue. They orchestrate the healing process.

mechanical loading: Contribution of mechanical forces, such as pressure, friction, and shear, that lead to the development of pressure ulcers.

Montgomery straps: Adhesive straps that can be applied to either side of a wound to provide a means of securing the dressing and subsequently change it without having to replace the tape each time.

muscle flap: Procedure in which a known muscle is moved along with its vascular supply (either intact or reestablished) into a defect.

musculocutaneous flap: Procedure in which a muscle combined with a portion of overlying skin and its intact vascular supply are moved. The portion of skin overlying the muscle is fed by perforators within the muscle.

necrobiosis lipodica diabeticum: Skin disease common in diabetics that is characterized by gradual degeneration and swelling of connective and elastic tissue with skin discoloration.

necrosis: Death of tissue.

necrotic tissue: Dead, devitalized, or avascular tissue.

neovascularization: Development of new blood vessels.

nonblanchable erythema: See *erythema.*

off-loading: Removal of pressure from a wound site.

operative repair: In the context of pressure ulcer repair, a variety of surgical procedures designed to repair pressure ulcers.

osteomyelitis: Inflammation of the bone marrow and adjacent bone, commonly due to infection.

overlay: See *support surfaces.*

partial thickness: Tissue destruction through the epidermis extending into, but not through, the dermis.

periulcer: Around the ulcer.

periwound: Skin or area directly around the wound.

pressure (interface): Force per unit area that acts perpendicularly between the body and the support surface. This parameter is affected by the stiffness of the support surface, the composition of the body tissue, and the geometry of the body being supported.

pressure reduction: Reduction of interface pressure, not necessarily below the level required to close capillaries.

pressure relief: Reduction of interface pressure below capillary-closing pressure.

pressure ulcer: Area of localized tissue damage usually located over a bony prominence that is caused by ischemia due to pressure. Pressure ulcers are many times referred to as "decubitus ulcers," "pressure sores," and "bed sores." These ulcers are staged according to the degree of tissue damage that is observed.

prevalence: Number of cases present in a population at one point in time.

primary intention healing: Closure and healing of a sutured wound.

psi (pounds per square inch): In wound care, this is the pressure exerted by a stream of fluid against one square inch of skin or wound surface.

purulent discharge: Product of inflammation that contains pus-cells (leukocytes and bacteria) and liquefied necrotic debris.

pyoderma gangrenosum: Rare, chronic, inflammatory disease that can cause painful distinctive lesions anywhere on the body but most commonly appear on the trunk and lower extremities.

radiant heat therapy: Type of adjunctive wound care therapy based on the premise that wounds are hypothermic and the healing is accelerated when wounds are warmed to the body's core temperature.

Raynaud's disease: Peripheral vascular disorder characterized by abnormal vasoconstriction of the extremities when exposed to cold or emotional stress.

reactive hyperemia: Reddening of the skin caused by blood rushing back into ischemic tissue.

rubor: Redness; one of the four classic signs of inflammation.

scab: Dried exudate covering a superficial wound.

secondary intention healing: Closure and healing of a wound by the formation of granulation tissue and epithelialization.

sensate flap: Procedure in which muscle, skin, and a sensory nerve are moved. The sensory nerve provides feeling to the flap.

seroma: Accumulation of fluid that is noted to build up at the incision site.

shear: Trauma caused by tissue layers sliding against each other; results in the disruption or strangulation of blood vessels. It is the mechanical force that acts on a unit area of skin in a direction parallel to the body's surface.

sickle cell anemia: Chronic, hereditary anemia in which crescent-shaped mature red blood cells are present.

sinus tract: Course or pathway that can extend in any direction from the wound surface; results in dead space with potential for abscess formation.

skin flap: Procedure in which a section of skin and associated subcutaneous tissue are moved from one part of the body to another, with the vascular supply maintained for nourishment. The vascular attachment can be the original vessel, rotated along with the flap, changed from one part of the flap to another, or reestablished by microvascular anastomoses once it has been placed in the new location.

skin graft: Procedure in which a segment of the dermis and epidermis are moved. The graft is completely separated from its blood supply and donor site and moved to a recipient site. A skin graft contains varying portions of epidermis and dermis. It can be full thickness or partial thickness, depending upon how much dermis is included in the graft.

skin strip: Removal of the epidermis by mechanical means.

slough: Moist, loose, stringy necrotic tissue.

support surfaces: Special beds, mattresses, mattress overlays, or seat cushions that reduce or relieve pressure while sitting or lying. Examples include

    air-flotation bed: Generic descriptor for low-air-loss beds and air-fluidized beds.

    air-fluidized bed: Class of support surfaces that uses a high rate of air flow to fluidize fine particulate material (such as sand or silicone beads) to produce a support medium that has characteristics similar to a liquid.

    alternating-air mattress or overlay: Mattress or overlay with interconnecting air cells that cyclically inflate and deflate to produce alternating high and low pressure intervals. Air cells with larger depth and diameter produce greater pressure relief over the body.

    donut-type device: Rigid, ring-shaped device created to relieve pressure on the sitting surface. This device is not recommended. Even though pressure is relieved on the tissue over the center of the ring, pressure in the tissue resting directly on the ring causes vascular congestion and may impede circulation to the tissues.

    dynamic device: Pressure-reducing device designed to change its support characteristics in a cyclical fashion. Examples include alternating-air mattresses and mechanical seats that change shape and redistribute pressure.

    foam mattress overlay: Thick foam slab with a textured surface designed to be placed on top of a standard hospital mattress to reduce pressure by enveloping the body. Its effectiveness is influenced by its thickness, density, and stiffness.

    kinetic therapy: Support surfaces designed to counteract problems with immobility by continuous passive motion or oscillation therapy. Kinetic therapy is also referred to as continuous lateral rotation therapy.

    low-air-loss bed: Series of interconnected woven fabric air pillows that allow some air to escape through the support surface. The pillows can be variably inflated to adjust the level of pressure relief.

    mattress replacement system: Mattress with pressure-reducing or pressure-relieving features that can be placed on an existing bed frame.

    overlay: General term used to describe support surfaces placed on top of a standard hospital mattress.

static air mattress: Vinyl mattress overlay composed of interconnected air cells that, before use, are inflated with a blower. The shifting of air among the cells distributes pressure uniformly over the support area to create a flotation effect.

static device: Pressure-reducing device designed to provide support characteristics that remain constant. There is no cycling of the air throughout the system. Examples include foam overlays, cushions, and water mattresses.

static water mattress: Vinyl mattress or overlay composed of interconnected compartments that are filled with water to distribute pressure uniformly over the support surface to create a flotation effect.

tissue biopsy: Use of a sharp instrument to obtain a sample of skin, muscle, or bone.

tissue expansion: Surgical technique during which an expandable device is placed beneath viable skin. The device is expanded with serial injections of saline solution and, when the skin has stretched, it is moved to cover a nearby defect.

tissue load: Distribution of pressure, friction, and shear on tissue.

tumor: Swelling; one of the four classic signs of inflammation.

tunneling: A narrow passageway under the surface of the skin that is generally open at the skin level; however, most tunneling is not visible.

ultrasound: Use of high-frequency sound waves as an adjunctive wound care therapy to improve the wound healing rate.

undermining: Closed passageway under the surface of the skin that is open only at the skin surface. Generally it appears as an area of skin ulceration at the margins of the ulcer with skin overlying the area.

V-Y advancement: Procedure that derives its name from the appearance of the postoperative wound. After an incision is made in the shape of a "V," the apex of the "V" is closed by advancing the central portion. This leaves a scar that looks like a "Y."

vacuum-assisted wound closure: An adjunctive wound care therapy that relies on negative pressure being applied to the wound in order to improve granulation tissue, decrease interstitial edema, decrease bacterial counts, and assist in more uniform closure of wounds, also called negative-pressure wound closure.

venous stasis ulcer: Ulceration of the lower extremity caused by stasis of blood from venous hypertension.

wound base: Uppermost viable layer of wound; may be covered with slough or eschar.

wound margin: Rim or border of wound.

BIBLIOGRAPHY

Agency for Health Care Policy and Research (AHCPR). (1992). Pressure Ulcers in Adults: Prediction and Prevention. Clinical Practice Guideline Number 3, Pub. No. 92-0047. National Library of Medicine. Retrieved April 6, 2004 from http://hstat.nim.nih.gov/

Agency for Health Care Policy and Research (AHCPR). (1994). Treatment of Pressure Ulcers. Clinical Guideline Number 15, Pub. No. 95-0652. National Library of Medicine. Retrieved April 6, 2004 from http://hstat.nlm.nih.gov/

Balanced Budget Act of 1997, Medicare and Medicaid Provisions. Retrieved April 7, 2004 from http://www.hccs.com/articles/misc/BBA_97.pdf

Barber, L.A. (2002). Clean technique or sterile technique? Let's take a moment to think. *Journal of Wound, Ostomy, Continence Nursing, 29*(1), 29-32.

Bates-Jensen, B. (1990). Pressure Sore Status Tool.

Bertek Pharmaceuticals, Inc. (1995). *Pressure Ulcers: A Practical Nursing Reference for the Chronic Wound Care Environment.* Sugar Land, TX: Author.

Birke, J.A., Pavich, M.A., Patout, C.A., & Horswell, R. (2002). Comparison of forefoot ulcer healing using alternative off-loading methods in patients with diabetes mellitus. *Advances in Skin & Wound Care, 15*(5), 210-15.

Bonham, P.A., & Flemister, B.G. (2002). *Guideline for management of wounds in patients with lower-extremity arterial disease.* Glenview, IL: Wound, Ostomy, and Continence Nurses Society.

Bowker, J.H., & Pfeifer, M.A. (2001). *Levin and O'Neal's the diabetic foot* (6th ed.). St. Louis, MO: Mosby–Year Book.

Braden, B., & Bergstrom, N. (1988). *Braden Scale for Predicting Pressure Sore Risk.* Retrieved April 6, 2004 from http://www.bradenscale.com

Braden, B., & Bergstrom, N. (1996). Risk assessment and risk-based programs of prevention in various settings. *Ostomy/Wound Management, 42*(10A), 6S-12S.

Bryant, R. (2000). *Acute and chronic wounds: Nursing management* (2nd ed.). St. Louis, MO: Mosby–Year Book.

Carabasi, R., & Jarrell, B. (1991). *Surgery* (2nd ed.). Philadelphia, PA: Harwal Publishing.

Dorland's illustrated medical dictionary (30th ed.). (2003). Philadelphia: W.B. Saunders Co.

Foster, L., & Moore, P. (1998). Acute surgical wound care 1: an overview of treatment. *British Journal of Nursing, 7*(18), 1101-06.

Fowler, E. (1990). Chronic wounds: An overview. In D. Krooner (Ed.), *Chronic problem wounds.* King of Prussia, PA: Health Management Publications, Inc.

Han, S.S., & Homstedt, J.O. (1981). *Human microscopic anatomy.* New York, NY: McGraw-Hill Book Co.

Hess, C.T. (2002). *Clinical guide to wound care* (4th ed.). Springhouse, PA: Springhouse Corp.

Kominsky, S.J. (1994). *Medical and surgical management of the diabetic foot.* St. Louis, MO: C.V. Mosby.

Krasner, D., & Kane, D. (2001). *Chronic wound care—a clinical source book for healthcare professionals* (3rd ed.). Wayne, PA: Health Management Publications, Inc.

Levine, M. (1973). *Introduction to clinical nursing* (2nd ed.). Philadelphia: F. A. Davis Co.

MacDonald, J.M. (2001). Wound healing and lymphedema: A new look at an old problem. *Ostomy/Wound Management, 47*(4), 52-57.

Maklebust, J., & Sieggreen, M. (2001). *Pressure ulcers: Guidelines for prevention and management* (3rd ed.). Springhouse, PA: Springhouse Corp.

Milne, C.T., Corbett, L.Q., & Dubuc, D.L. (2003). *Wound, ostomy, and continence nursing secrets.* Philadephia: Hanley & Belfus, Inc.

Morison, M., & Moffatt, C. (1994). *A color guide to the nursing management of leg ulcers* (2nd ed.). London: Mosby.

Motta, G. (2003). *Kestrel wound product sourcebook, 2003-2004.* Kestrel Health Information, Inc: Bristol, VT.

Poore, S., Cameron, J., & Cherry, G. (2002). Venous leg ulcer recurrence: prevention and healing. *Journal of Wound Care, 11*(5):197-99.

Shea, J.D. (1975). Pressure sores: classification and management. *Clinical Orthopaedics and Related Research, 112*:89-100.

Stotts, N.A., Barbour, S., Griggs, K., Bouvier, B., Buhlman, L., Wipke-Tevis, D. et al. (1997). Sterile versus clean technique in postoperative wound care of patients with open surgical wounds: A pilot study. *Journal of Wound, Ostomy, Continence Nursing, 24*(1), 10-18.

Sussman, C., & Bates-Jensen, B. (2004). *Wound care: a collaborative practice manual for physical therapists and nurses.* Philadelphia: Lippincott Williams & Wilkins.

US Department of Health and Human Services. *Healthy People 2010.* Retrieved April 5, 2004 from http://www.healthypeople.gov/document/html/objectives/01-16.htm

Van Rijswijk, L. (1996). Wound care practices in the home: Signposts to effective patient outcomes. *Wound Care Policies & Procedures Manual,* (2nd ed.). Skillman, NJ: Convatec House Calls Total Wound Management Program.

Warriner, R.A., III. (2002, Nov. 7-8). *Exploring Advanced Technologies in Wound Management.* Presentation at Praxis Clinical Services Seminar, Las Vegas, NV.

Wise, L.C., Hoffman, J., Grant, L., & Bostrom, J. (1997). Nursing wound care survey: Sterile and nonsterile glove choice. *Journal of Wound, Ostomy, Continence Nursing, 24*(3), 144-50.

Wound, Ostomy, and Continence Nurses Society (WOCN). *Clinical Fact Sheet Quick Assessment of Leg Ulcers.* Retrieved April 6, 2004 from http://www.wocn.org

From Wound, Ostomy, and Continence Nurses Society (WOCN). *Professional Practice Fact Sheet. Medicare Part B Coverage for Support Surfaces in the Home Health Setting.* Retrieved April 7, 2004 from http://www.wocn.org/pdf/PARTB.pdf

Young, T., & Fowler, A. (1998). Nursing management of skin grafts and donor sites. *British Journal of Nursing, 7*(6), 324-28.

INDEX

patients
  education on pressure ulcers for, 60, 82-84
  with incontinence, 20, 66
  nutritional status of, 21-22, 51, 74, 75*fig*-77*fig*
  wounds of diabetic, 91*fig*, 94*fig*, 96*fig*-98
periwound erythema, 52*fig*
periwound injuries, 121-124
permeability, 14
PHMB (polyhexamethylene biguanide), 130
photographic documentation, 31, 33-34
positioning patients, 52-53
pressure, 19
Pressure Sore Status Tool, 67*fig*-68*fig*, 69*fig*-70*fig*
pressure ulcer formation
  causes of, 63-64
  common sites for, 65*fig*
  friction and, 65
  mechanism of pressure on skin/underlying structures
      and, 64*fig*
  moisture and, 66
  shearing and, 65
"Pressure Ulcer Prediction and Prevention Algorithm"
  (AHCPR), 47
pressure ulcers
  adjunctive therapies for, 80-81
  assessment and measurement of, 66-74
  care of, 79-80
  common sites for, 65*t*
  education on, 60, 82-84
  formation of, 63-66
  mechanical loading to prevent, 51-53, 58*fig*
  nutritional status and, 51, 74, 75*fig*-77*fig*
  operative repair of, 81-82
  photograph of, 64*fig*
  prediction and prevention algorithm for, 48*fig*
  risk assessment for, 48-51
  skin care and management of, 59-60
  stage III, 119*fig*
  stage III from prosthesis, 120*fig*
  support surfaces and, 53-57, 59
  tools used to assess, 48-49, 50*fig*
  treatment and prevention of, 74-79
pressure ulcers assessment
  nutritional status, 74, 75*fig*-77*fig*
  pressure sore status tools, 67*fig*-68*fig*, 68, 69*fig*-70*fig*
  staging of, 66, 71-74

pressure ulcer treatment
  adjunctive therapies, 80-81
  client education on, 82-84
  debridement, 79
  dressings, 79-80
  infection control, 80
  managing tissue loads and support surfaces, 77-79
  operative repair, 81-82
  wound cleansing, 79
primary closure, 12*fig*
proliferative phase, 15
proteins, 22
Pseudomonas species, 114-115
PSST (Pressure Sore Status Tool), 33
PUSH (Pressure Ulcer Scale for Healing), 33
PVD (peripheral vascular disease), 93, 95
pyridoxine, 21-22

Q
QI (quality improvement) measures for pressure ulcers,
  83-84

R
radiant heat therapy, 157
radiation therapy, 22
red wound classification, 30
reimbursement practices
  additional steps in successful, 163-165
  durable medical equipment regional carriers, 164*fig*
  importance of understanding, 161
  major payor mix and, 161-162
  of managed care/HMOs, 162
  of Medicaid/MediCal programs, 162
  of Medicare, 162-163
  See also Medicare
reticular dermis, 4
rh-PDGF-BB (becaplermin), 154
riboflavin, 21-22
right hip incision primary closure, 12*fig*
risk assessment for pressure ulcer
  Braden scale, 49, 50*fig*
  education on, 60
  health care team members performing, 49, 51
  mechanical loading and, 51-53
  nutrition and, 51
  prevention algorithm and, 48*fig*
  skin care and management, 59-60
  support surfaces, 53-59
  timing of, 51
  tools used for, 48-49
  variables associated with, 48

PRETEST KEY

Wound Management and Healing

1.	b	Chapter 1
2.	a	Chapter 1
3.	c	Chapter 2
4.	b	Chapter 2
5.	d	Chapter 3
6.	a	Chapter 3
7.	c	Chapter 4
8.	c	Chapter 4
9.	b	Chapter 4
10.	a	Chapter 4
11.	d	Chapter 6
12.	b	Chapter 6
13.	c	Chapter 6
14.	a	Chapter 7
15.	c	Chapter 8
16.	c	Chapter 8
17.	d	Chapter 8
18.	b	Chapter 9
19.	b	Chapter 10
20.	c	Chapter 10
21.	a	Chapter 10
22.	c	Chapter 11
23.	c	Chapter 12
24.	d	Chapter 13

Notes

Notes

Notes

Notes

Notes

Western Schools® offers over 2,000 hours to suit all your interests – and requirements!

Cardiovascular
Cardiovascular Nursing: A Comprehensive Overview ....32 hrs
Cardiovascular Pharmacology...11 hrs
A The 12-Lead ECG in Acute Coronary Syndromes ....42 hrs

Clinical Conditions/Nursing Practice
A Advanced Assessment...35 hrs
Airway Management with a Tracheal Tube ....1 hr
Asthma: Nursing Care Across the Lifespan ....28 hrs
Auscultation Skills...38 hrs
— Heart Sounds ....20 hrs
— Breath Sounds ....18 hrs
Chest Tube Management...2 hrs
Clinical Care of the Diabetic Foot ....8 hrs
A Complete Nurses Guide to Diabetes Care.....................................37 hrs
Diabetes Essentials for Nurses ....30 hrs
Death, Dying & Bereavement ....30 hrs
Essentials of Patient Education ....30 hrs
Healing Nutrition ....24 hrs
Holistic & Complementary Therapies ....18 hrs
Home Health Nursing (2nd ed.) ....30 hrs
Humor in Healthcare: The Laughter Prescription ....20 hrs
Orthopedic Nursing: Caring for Patients with
Musculoskeletal Disorders ....30 hrs
Osteomyelitis..2 hrs
Pain & Symptom Management...1 hr
Pain Management: Principles and Practice ....30 hrs
A Palliative Practices: An Interdisciplinary Approach ....66 hrs
— Issues Specific to Palliative Care............................20 hrs
— Specific Disease States and Symptom
Management ....24 hrs
— The Dying Process, Grief, and Bereavement. ....22 hrs
Pharmacologic Management of Asthma...1 hr
Seizures: A Basic Overview ....1 hr
The Neurological Exam ....1 hr
Wound Management and Healing ....30 hrs

Critical Care/ER/OR
Basic Nursing of Head, Chest, Abdominal, Spine
and Orthopedic Trauma..20 hrs
Cosmetic Breast Surgery ....1 hr
A Case Studies in Critical Care Nursing...46 hrs
Critical Care & Emergency Nursing ....30 hrs
Hemodynamic Monitoring ....18 hrs
A Nurse Anesthesia...58 hrs
— Common Diseases ....20 hrs
— Common Procedures ....21 hrs
— Drugs ....17 hrs
A Practical Guide to Moderate Sedation/Analgesia ....31 hrs
Principles of Basic Trauma Nursing ....30 hrs
Weight Loss Surgery: A Treatment for Morbid Obesity ....1 hr

Geriatrics
Alzheimer's Disease: A Complete Guide for Nurses ....25 hrs
Nursing Care of the Older Adult ....30 hrs
Psychosocial Issues Affecting Older Adults ....16 hrs

Infectious Diseases/Bioterrorism
Avian Influenza..1 hr
Biological Weapons..5 hrs
Bioterrorism & the Nurse's Response to WMD ....5 hrs
Bioterrorism Readiness: The Nurse's Critical Role ....2 hrs
Hepatitis C: The Silent Killer (2nd ed.) ....3 hrs
HIV/AIDS ....1 or 2 hrs
Infection Control Training for Healthcare Workers ....4 hrs
Influenza: A Vaccine-Preventable Disease ....1 hr
MRSA ....1 hr
Pertussis: Diagnosis, Treatment, and Prevention ....3 hrs
Smallpox ....2 hrs
Tuberculosis Across the Lifespan ....3 hrs
West Nile Virus (2nd ed.) ....1 hr

Oncology
Cancer in Women ....30 hrs
Cancer Nursing (2nd ed.) ....36 hrs
Chemotherapy and Biotherapies ....10 hrs

Pediatrics/Maternal-Child/Women's Health
A Assessment and Care of the Well Newborn ....34 hrs
Diabetes in Children ....30 hrs
End-of-Life Care for Children and Their Families ....2 hrs
Induction of Labor...8 hrs
Manual of School Health ....30 hrs
Maternal-Newborn Nursing ....30 hrs
Menopause: Nursing Care for Women Throughout Mid-Life ......25 hrs
A Obstetric and Gynecologic Emergencies ....44 hrs
— Obstetric Emergencies....................................22 hrs
— Gynecologic Emergencies................................22 hrs
Pediatric Nursing: Routine to Emergent Care..............................30 hrs
Pediatric Pharmacology ....10 hrs
Pediatric Physical Assessment ....10 hrs
A Practice Guidelines for Pediatric Nurse Practitioners ....46 hrs
Respiratory Diseases in the Newborn ....3 hrs
Women's Health: Contemporary Advances and Trends (3rd ed.) ..24 hrs

Professional Issues/Management/Law
Documentation for Nurses ....24 hrs
Medical Error Prevention: Patient Safety ....2 hrs
Management and Leadership in Nursing ....20 hrs
Ohio Law: Standards of Safe Nursing Practice (4th ed.) ....1 hr
Surviving and Thriving in Nursing ....30 hrs
Understanding Managed Care...30 hrs

Psychiatric/Mental Health
A ADHD in Children and Adults ....8 hrs
Attention Deficit Hyperactivity Disorders
Throughout the Lifespan..30 hrs
Basic Psychopharmacology ....5 hrs
Behavioral Approaches to Treating Obesity ....13 hrs
A Bipolar Disorder ....10 hrs
A Child/Adolescent Clinical Psychopharmacology ....12 hrs
A Childhood Maltreatment ....10 hrs
A Clinical Psychopharmacology ....10 hrs
A Collaborative Therapy with Multi-stressed Families ....30 hrs
Depression: Prevention, Diagnosis, and Treatment.......................25 hrs
A Ethnicity and the Dementias ....25 hrs
A Evidence-Based Mental Health Practice ....22 hrs
A Geropsychiatric and Mental Health Nursing..............................40 hrs
A Growing Up with Autism ....21 hrs
A Integrating Traditional Healing Practices into Counseling ....35 hrs
A Integrative Treatment for Borderline Personality Disorder ....21 hrs
IPV (Intimate Partner Violence) (2nd ed.) ....1 or 3 hrs
A Mental Disorders in Older Adults ....25 hrs
A Mindfulness and Psychotherapy ....25 hrs
A Multicultural Perspectives in Working with Families ....27 hrs
A Obsessive Compulsive Disorder ....9 hrs
A Problem and Pathological Gambling ....9 hrs
Psychiatric Nursing: Current Trends in Diagnosis ....30 hrs
Psychiatric Principles & Applications ....30 hrs
A Psychosocial Adjustment to Chronic Illness in
Children and Adolescents ....8 hrs
A Schizophrenia ....5 hrs
Substance Abuse ....32 hrs
Suicide...21 hrs
A Trauma Therapy ....11 hrs
A Treating Explosive Kids ....14 hrs
A Treating Substance Use Problems in Psychotherapy Practice ......24 hrs
A Treating Victims of Mass Disaster and Terrorism.......................6 hrs

REV. 09/03/08